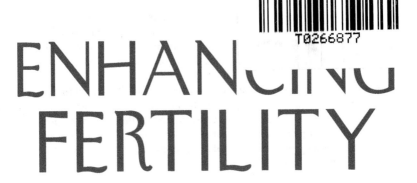

ENHANCING FERTILITY

A Couple's Guide
to Natural Approaches

CHRIS D. MELETIS, N.D.,
& LIZ BROWN

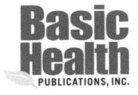

Basic Health
PUBLICATIONS, INC.

The information contained in this book is based upon the research and personal and professional experiences of the authors. It is not intended as a substitute for consulting with your physician or other healthcare provider. Any attempt to diagnose and treat an illness should be done under the direction of a healthcare professional.

The publisher does not advocate the use of any particular healthcare protocol but believes the information in this book should be available to the public. The publisher and authors are not responsible for any adverse effects or consequences resulting from the use of the suggestions, preparations, or procedures discussed in this book. Should the reader have any questions concerning the appropriateness of any procedures or preparation mentioned, the authors and the publisher strongly suggest consulting a professional healthcare advisor.

Basic Health Publications, Inc.

Library of Congress Cataloging-in-Publication Data

Meletis, Chris D.

   Enhancing fertility : a couple's guide to natural approaches / Chris
D. Meletis, N.D., and Liz Brown.
      p. cm.
   Includes bibliographical references and index.
   ISBN 978-1-59120-054-3 (Pbk.)
   ISBN 978-1-68162-715-1 (Hardcover)

   1. Infertility—Alternative treatment. 2. Naturopathy. I. Brown,
Liz, 1971– II. Title.

   RC889.M3793   2004
   616.6'9206—dc22

                                        2004007263

Editor: Susan E. Davis
Typesetting/Book design: Gary A. Rosenberg
Cover design: Mike Stromberg

Contents

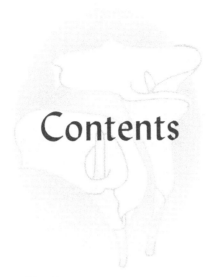

Acknowledgments

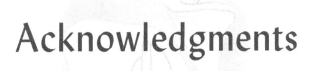

First and foremost I would like to thank God, for His creative power and the magnificent gifts He has given humanity. May His wisdom bless each couple that reads this book and seeks the joy of parenthood.

A special note to my wonderful wife: You are the best life partner I could have ever imagined. To my boys, Nicholas and Matthew, you helped inspire this book, for you each give me an appreciation of the blessing of parenthood. And finally, to our unborn baby whom we never got to know on earth, we eagerly await the ultimate of family unions for all of eternity.

—Chris D. Meletis, N.D.

I would like to thank my parents, Don and Barb Brown, for giving me the gift of life and for their ongoing encouragement, love, and patience. Many thanks also to my brother, Jeff, and my friends, and special thanks to Dominic Orlando for his help with graphics. I would like to dedicate this book in memory of Sverre Peter Roang, a dear friend and mentor, whose tireless dedication to peace, promoting natural foods, questioning authority, and enthusiasm for life inspire me every day.

—Liz Brown

Special thanks to Norman Goldfind and Susan E. Davis for their support, hard work, and sharing the belief that natural medicine can serve as the key to unlocking and unleashing vibrant health in the pursuit of enhanced fertility.

Contributors

Owen K. Davis, M.D.

Catherine Downey, N.D.

Rosetta Koach, L.M.T., N.D.

Peter N. Kolettis, M.D.

Zalman Levine, M.D.

Robert K. McLellan, M.D., M.P.H.

Susan Roberts, N.D.

David Russ, D.C.

Tamara L. Staudt, N.D., M.S.O.M.

Lucy Vaughters, P.A.C., C.C.H.

Werner Vosloo, M.Sc.Hom.

Philip Werthman, M.D.

Shaun C. Williams, M.D.

Glenn Zielinski, D.C.

Katherine Zieman, N.D.

Haosheng Zhang, M.S.O.M, Lac.

Guanying Zhou, M.S.O.M., Lac.

Introduction

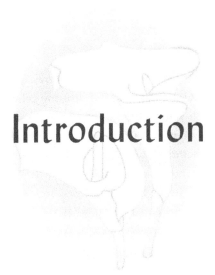

This book is dedicated to the millions of couples who have faced the challenge of trying to get pregnant. Our goal is simple: to provide you with a clear guide of do's and don'ts that can swing the odds in your favor, with a focus on natural, safe, well-researched therapeutic and preventive approaches.

Your journey toward enhanced fertility has just begun. The first step is taking charge of your destiny by seeking the knowledge you need to boost your fertility. This book will help you do just that. Your fertility as a couple depends on the sum total of both positive and negative variables related to your health. Understanding what those variables are and making healthy choices as a result will help the two of you increase your odds of getting pregnant and giving birth to a healthy baby.

Maybe you're about to start trying to conceive for the first time and you're taking extra care to learn as much as you can beforehand. Or perhaps you've been trying to get pregnant for a while without success. Doctors may have told you there's no hope that you will. While that is certainly true for some people, the majority of infertile couples can overcome obstacles to conception and eventually become parents. In some situations—for example, in the case of anatomical abnormalities and blockage of reproductive system ducts—surgery or other high-tech procedures may be necessary to accomplish that goal. And, unfortunately, it is true that not everyone can overcome infertility.

But when it comes to many causes of infertility—hormonal imbalances and poor sperm quality among them—healthy diet and lifestyle choices and natural medicine can often enhance fertility significantly. Nutritional, environmental, and botanical medicine, as well as traditional Chinese medicine and homeopathy, all have something to offer. Testifying to this great news are the exciting research reports and success stories of happy couples who have overcome infertility naturally that you'll read about throughout this book. Barring physical problems beyond your control, you have the power to take charge of your health and, in doing so, to boost your fertility.

Striving to get pregnant can be stressful, and stress itself can alter some couples' ability to conceive. Rather than allowing stress to get the best of you, take this opportunity to grow with your partner as you embark on this quest together. So often in our society, the woman is blamed for being unable to conceive or carry a baby to term, but male factors account for a large share of infertility, too. Even so, useful resources for men about how to enhance their fertility naturally have been sorely lacking—until now. In the following pages, both you and your partner will find a wealth of information and tips on what you can do—individually and together—to fully realize your fertility potential. As with any successful team, if one player needs more assistance, the other player's role is to pitch in and work for mutual victory. In addition to being emotionally supportive of the partner experiencing a fertility challenge (and bear in mind that sometimes both partners contribute to infertility), the other partner should strive to reach his or her peak fertility through healthy diet and lifestyle choices to boost the couple's overall odds of conceiving.

If you aren't experiencing a fertility challenge and you just want to fine-tune your system as you attempt to get pregnant and bring a healthy baby to term, this book is also for you. Being as healthy as possible will improve your chances of achieving that goal. If you are among the one in six couples considered infertile at one time or another, paying special attention to the advice, research, and common sense shared in this book can help shift things in the right direction for you and your loved one. Regardless of the reason you've picked up this book, the reality is that it is designed for those desperately seeking enhanced fertility. But it is also useful as a guide to better health for a lifetime, independent of age or fertility goals.

As we review the various aspects of enhancing fertility in the chapters that follow, the pearls of clinical and practical wisdom also apply to your overall health. The healthier you make your body, the greater the likelihood the seed of life will find fertile soil and flourish. Our intent is to provide useful information for you to share with each other and with your physician as you incorporate what's appropriate for your individual needs.

Blessings to you and your partner as you seek the ultimate of all gifts—the baby you both want so much.

1

Building a Foundation of Health

As you have probably already discovered, getting pregnant isn't always that easy. It can be a very complex process, and many variables have to be in place for it to happen. Our goal is to empower you and your partner by providing useful information to make the process less complicated and to help you get pregnant.

Let's start with the basics: To get pregnant, a woman has to ovulate and release an egg, or ovum. A man has to produce enough normal sperm that can move well. Then he must be able to ejaculate sperm that can make their way through the woman's reproductive system to reach and fertilize the ovum. In turn, the ovum has to be able to develop and implant itself in the endometrium (the lining of the uterus), where it can develop into a healthy baby over the next nine months. Refer to Figure 1.1 on page 4 and Figure 1.2 on page 5 for illustrations of the male and female reproductive systems.

Considering all the physiological factors necessary to establish a pregnancy, it's really not surprising that roughly 6 million Americans are infertile at one time or another. That means they have been unable to conceive after at least one year of regular intercourse without contraceptive use. Fertility declines as we age (especially after age thirty-five for women), so people who wait until later in life to conceive may find it particularly challenging. That means they may need to enhance their bodies' fertility to make it happen.

About 25 percent of infertility cases are related to a problem with ovarian function and ovulation in the woman. Another 25 percent are due to a problem with the woman's Fallopian tubes. Male causes—such as low sperm production, obstruction of the duct that carries the ejaculate fluid, abnormal semen, and immunity-related factors—account for at least one-quarter of cases. (Some estimate the percentage of male causes as closer to one-third or even approaching one-half of all causes, though estimates vary.) Seventeen percent of cases are unexplained, and the female reproductive disease endometriosis or other assorted

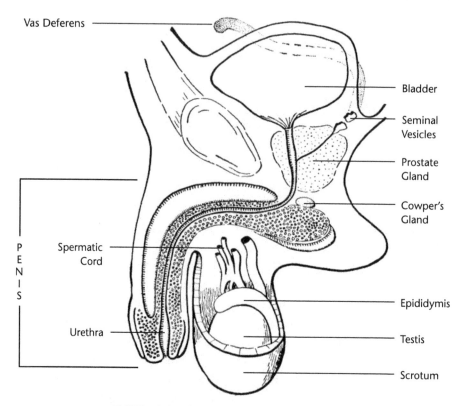

FIGURE 1.1. The Male Reproductive System

causes account for the remainder. *Primary infertility* is defined as infertility without any previous pregnancy. *Secondary infertility* refers to a case in which there has been a previous pregnancy.

It takes two to tango for many things in life, and this is especially so when it comes to getting pregnant. Sometimes we take for granted just how much healthy partnership the process requires.

YOU HAVE THE POWER TO ENHANCE YOUR FERTILITY

The great news is that many couples are able to enhance their fertility while building better health for themselves. That's because a combination of environmental, nutritional, and lifestyle factors can be altered to boost a couple's ability to conceive. It's simple: Adopting healthy habits can increase your odds of becoming a parent. In fact, natural medicine is backed by an impressive body of research and has a rich history of treating infertility effectively with herbs and other gentle treatments, like acupuncture, that you'll learn about later in the book.

Throughout this guide for couples, you'll find out how to make your bodies as fertile as they can be with natural approaches. The first few chapters will help you build a healthy foundation by eating well, avoiding environmental toxins, knowing when to conceive, and undergoing routine medical tests to determine if any problems exist that need to be resolved. Later chapters will address specific problems that can cause infertility in men and women and explain how natural medicine—botanical and nutritional medicine, homeopathy, physical medicine, and classical and traditional Chinese medicine (CCM and TCM)—can often help couples overcome infertility.

It makes sense that cultivating good health would increase your odds of getting pregnant. It's analogous to another process in nature: raising a garden. Before putting seeds in the ground, it's important to choose a plot with rich soil, where plants will most likely thrive. The seeds must be of high quality to ensure that the fruits, vegetables, or flowers they produce are robust. A plant in an empty lot full of garbage and debris that doesn't have enough water, light, and nutrients may survive for a while—perhaps throughout an entire growing season—but what little it yields will be of poor quality.

Tending one's internal garden to create the best environment where the seed of life grows is paramount in becoming as fertile as you can be. Being well nourished and adaptive when it comes to dealing with environmental challenges—that is, overcoming them with acquired coping skills or, better yet, avoiding them—is essential for a healthy garden and a healthy body. Learning how to avoid and cope with overt mental and physical stressors like office conflicts, nutrient deficiencies,

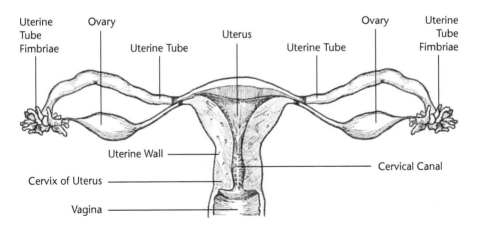

FIGURE 1.2. The Female Reproductive System

poor lifestyle habits, environmental toxins, and medications that compromise some aspect of health will help you achieve an optimal state of health and fertility.

Let's be clear: It's not your fault if you haven't been making the best decisions possible for your health. We live in a society that requires very active and informed decisions to avoid the pitfalls that trap the vast majority. That's why we're going to give you the edge that can help you find the "fertile zone."

HOW MUCH DO YOU VALUE YOUR HEALTH?

As you read the following chapters, you'll discover that by improving your health, you increase your chances of enjoying a higher quality of life, greater satisfaction from life, and in many cases, increased fertility. We strongly encourage you to complete the following exercise before reading the rest of this book.

Clear your mind for a moment, and if your partner is around have him or her sit down with you and read this aloud. On a scale of one to ten, where are you on the Health Value Index? This index reflects how important health maintenance is to you. One equals "I need not worry about my body, it really doesn't matter what I do, life goes on and I can always fix things once something goes wrong." On the opposite end of the spectrum, ten equals "My body is my temple, and what I eat and do to my body directly affect my immediate and long-term health; thus I am active in my health journey."

Pick the number from one to ten that most reflects how you value your health. Now it's time for a challenge—to see how truly aware you are about the effort you put into staying well and improving your physical health.

The Automobile Analogy

Cars come with owner's manuals that tell us how to take care of them and get as much performance from them as possible. Among the usual recommendations are oil changes every 3,000 to 5,000 miles, regular tune-ups, tire rotations, air filter changes, using a certain grade of gasoline, taking care of the engine, and so on. Our bodies deserve even better care than our cars, yet they don't come with an owner's manual, and we often take their maintenance for granted.

Let's take a brief look at how maintenance checks for cars are analogous to health maintenance for you and your partner. Oil changes can be equated to making sure that you are drinking enough water, that your bowels are working well, and that your engine is lubricated properly to prevent undue wear and tear. This includes making sure you have sufficient antioxidants (food-based protective molecules that you'll read about later in this chapter) to defend against disease-causing agents called free radicals, which are produced by chemicals, other environmental factors, and even regular metabolism. Think of antioxidants like the additives you put in your engine oil: they prevent undue wear and tear to the body.

Tune-ups for the body are similar to those for a car. We perform routine maintenance on cars in the hope that smaller expenses for proper upkeep will help us avoid the big bill of a breakdown. The investment of going to your physician or other healthcare provider to make sure everything is working well should occur yearly, regardless of whether or not you have specific health concerns. Proper diagnostic work, including routine, complete blood work, will help make sure your engine is not misfiring. If your car is worthy of being hooked up to a computer to see how it's performing, so are you. The strategy is to go to your doctor *before* your body breaks down. However, some breakdowns in our bodies can't be predicted and are often irreparable. Whatever you do with your car or your body, you *never* want to violate the warranty that your car or body comes with. Replacement parts for your body are hard to come by, so take good care of the originals.

Rotating the tires on a car is analogous to making sure you're keeping in shape so you can keep rolling. It's easy to let exercise drop off the priority list when our lives get hectic, but don't underestimate the importance of physical activity; it is a crucial variable in the equation for good health.

Just as we regularly change the air filter on our cars, we should also take care to make sure we're not loading our bodies down with dangerous chemicals, cigarette smoke, alcohol, or other things that are likely to smother us with signs and symptoms of impurity and excess toxicity, compromising health and sometimes overwhelming our system.

Let's look at fuel quality. Imagine this scenario: Gas prices are going up, and there's a very convenient neighborhood station selling gas for 99 cents a gallon. It strikes you as a bargain you can't pass up. But this is an off-brand gas station known for providing inferior fuel, so long-term bad effects are associated with filling up at this station. Would you risk your investment in your car for a little savings? Most people would agree it isn't worth the risk. Yet how often do we stop by the fast-food drive-through for that 99-cent bargain, even though everywhere we turn—the medical establishment, the media, conversations with friends and family—there's strong evidence that fast food is bad for us. Isn't it strange how we often think more about our cars, which last a decade or two at best, when we need to rely on our bodies *literally* for a lifetime? We can't trade in our bodies (not yet, at least); therefore, we have to do our best to keep them functioning optimally so we can enjoy healthy, happy, long lives.

One aspect of human health that has no automobile counterpart is emotional health. Keeping stress in check and feeling happy and satisfied with your life and your relationships with family, friends, and spouses can do wonders for your health on both an emotional and a physical level. Being emotionally healthy will make you a better parent, too.

Did that discussion influence your place on the Health Value Index? What is your number now? What is your partner's number now?

More Important Than a Trip to the Dentist

Most of us have been well trained to visit our dentist on a fairly routine basis, and if we forget, the dentist is almost certainly going to remind us with a postcard in the mail. It's great that we care so much about our teeth; after all, a pretty smile, healthy gums, and strong teeth to chew with are important. Visiting the dentist regularly is one of the best models for disease prevention and health maintenance in the world.

Think of it this way: You go to the dentist every six months to a year. During the visit, you recline in a chair in a very compromising and vulnerable position, a bright light shining in your eyes, with a relative stranger putting his or her fingers in your mouth and using drills, picks, scrapers, and odd-flavored solutions to promote your oral health. Best of all, you get to drool publicly. It's not exactly a great time, but we do it anyway because we know we should. So why do most of us spend much less time maintaining our overall health? Keeping healthy usually entails less unsavory measures, such as eating healthy, tasty organic food, enjoying fresh air and nature on brisk walks, and taking time to relax. Going to the doctor isn't always pleasant; it can be downright uncomfortable, and sometimes even painful. But the question is simple: Do you pay as much attention to the rest of your body as you do to your mouth? What if in your later years you're driving around in a well-maintained car, with a winning smile, but falling apart otherwise? The image would be funny if it weren't so sad.

Baby on Board

There are many benefits of achieving the best possible state of health prior to conception. Healthy women are better prepared to handle nine months of pregnancy, should it occur. It is more likely that a baby on board will develop normally when supplied with the right nutrients from the mother. For example, inadequate maternal intake of folic acid can result in neural tube defects in the fetus. Sufficient iron intake is needed to create a healthy blood supply for the baby, and vitamin B_6 is crucial for neurological development.

A pregnancy is like a long road trip, with physical and physiological mountains to climb. Think about it: You wouldn't set off on a cross-country trip from New

York to California without making sure your car was in good operating shape, that it had a fresh oil change, plenty of gas in the tank, and good rubber on the wheels. Likewise, couples preparing for the journey of parenthood should have thorough physical exams and be disease-free and properly nourished before the trip and along the way. After reading this book, you'll understand how to determine and improve your health status, what physical tests your doctor should conduct for you, which questionnaires can help you gauge your own nutritional intake, and what recommendations to follow to improve your health. Doing all those things will make the road trip smoother and more enjoyable.

Another side benefit of improving your health is that when the baby arrives, you will be more likely to have the energy and ability to fully experience the joy of your new child. Parenthood is a long and exciting journey that begins at conception. You might as well gear up for it by taking exceptional care of yourselves starting now.

FEEDING FERTILITY

Giving your body the right nutrients, in the right amounts, is key to making your body as fertile as possible. Much research has proven that inadequate intake of specific vitamins, minerals, and amino acids can compromise fertility in men and women. Antioxidants, including vitamins C and E, zinc, and selenium, are especially important.

The body needs antioxidants to fight free radicals, which are molecules that damage healthy cells in the body as they search for electrons to stabilize themselves. This damage is called *free-radical oxidation*. Free radicals are found in cigarette smoke and air pollution and can result from too much sun exposure, but they are also natural byproducts of metabolism and are used by the body to fend off attacking germs. Getting enough antioxidants in the diet and via supplements helps build up the body's defense against free-radical damage, protecting cells from their deleterious effects.

Sperm, like other cells, are vulnerable to free-radical damage. This is partly because they have membranes that are rich in lipids, or fats, which are very susceptible to oxidative damage called *lipid peroxidation*. In one study, high free-radical activity in the male reproductive tract was linked to infertility in 40 percent of male subjects.[1] Adequate antioxidants protect sperm, allowing them to function normally and increasing the chance that they will make it to their destination in the female reproductive tract—the Fallopian tubes. When healthy sperm arrive at a fertile and developed ovum and the timing is right, the magical moment of conception occurs.

Fertility-Friendly Nutrients

Vitamin E has been shown to protect sperm from lipid peroxidation in the cell membrane that impairs sperm motility (the ability of sperm to move well). In a 1996 study reported in the *Journal of Andrology,* subjects with defective sperm motility who took oral vitamin E experienced decreased lipid peroxidation in sperm and improved motility.[2] Even more encouraging in the study was the finding that eleven of the fifty-two patients who took vitamin E impregnated their spouses. Nine of the pregnancies resulted in normal-term deliveries. You'll learn more about the benefits of vitamin E in Chapters 2 and 8.

Vitamin C is another antioxidant nutrient that plays a role in fertility. Semen contains a high concentration of vitamin C (also called ascorbic acid). In semen, this antioxidant vitamin helps maintain the genetic integrity of sperm cells by protecting their DNA (genetic material) from oxidative damage.[3]

Depleted levels of vitamin C have also contributed to death of the corpus luteum in female research animals.[4] The corpus luteum is the mature ovarian follicle that ruptures to expel a potential mature ovum, or egg. Other animal studies have found that high doses of vitamins C and E fed to female mice partially prevented an age-related reduction in ovulation rate.[5] Though we shouldn't assume that results in humans would necessarily mimic these findings, they do hint at the potential for such vitamins to enhance human fertility. You'll see, as you read on, that it's easy to consume enough vitamin C through diet and vitamin supplements to promote reproductive health.

Minerals play a major role in fertility, too. Humans need adequate zinc and selenium to optimize the odds of conceiving. Zinc, along with folic acid, is involved in synthesizing DNA and RNA. In men, zinc deficiency leads to decreased spermatogenesis, or sperm formation, and impaired fertility.[6] In women, supplementation with zinc has been shown to reverse low female fertility.[7] Pregnant women need plenty of zinc, too. Fortunately, preventing or reversing a zinc deficiency is relatively easy with supplementation and a good diet. Iodine, chromium, selenium, coenzyme Q_{10}, arginine, and carnitine are among the other fertility-friendly nutrients that will be discussed in upcoming chapters.

Dietary Do's and Don'ts

While vitamins and minerals positively affect fertility, some dietary items actually keep sperm cell membranes from functioning well. Fortunately, you can control what you put in your mouth once you know what to avoid. Omega-6 polyunsaturated fats like safflower, corn, and sunflower oils, for example, are notorious for causing oxidative damage when overconsumed. If you consume too many of these kinds of fats, the body oxidizes them and they become free radicals, potentially causing harm to your cells and leading to a wide array of health problems. Taking vitamin E supplements can help prevent oxidation of omega-6 polyunsaturated fats, while moderating your intake of these fats is helpful, too. It's best also to limit your intake of saturated fats, including animal fats and coconut and palm oils, as well as trans-fatty acids (produced when heating and frying with cooking oil), partially hydrogenated oil (found in most processed foods like chips, cookies, and crackers), and cottonseed oil (which contains gossypol, a substance proven to decrease sperm function). Steering clear of these is beneficial to the heart and your overall health, too.

Healthy alternatives to bad fats include oils high in essential fatty acids (EFAs). They are called essential because the body can't make them on its own, and it's essential to consume them in the diet. In unoxidized form, EFAs, which include omega-3 and omega-6 fatty acids, improve sperm quality and function, since they are organic components of sperm cell membranes. Borage, black currant, flaxseed, evening primrose, and fish oils are some sources of these beneficial fats. (Note, however, that excessive intake of omega-6s can be deleterious.)

A diet high in antioxidants from fresh fruits and vegetables (ideally, organic ones) is best. Eating whole grains, good fats, and less refined and processed foods helps set the stage for conception. A healthy diet also decreases the chances of developing gestational diabetes, a form of diabetes that sets in during pregnancy.

As you'll read in the following chapters, maintaining a healthy weight by eating well and exercising moderately is ideal for conceiving, too. Being excessively underweight or overweight can decrease your odds of getting pregnant. Studies have shown that women who have anorexia nervosa and other eating disorders sometimes face extra challenges with fertility and reproduction.[8] Athletes who train rigorously, ballet dancers, and women who diet excessively sometimes stop menstruating, disrupting their natural ability to reproduce. Adopting a moderate exercise program and eating enough nutrient-dense foods are positive steps toward increasing fertility and the odds of having a healthy pregnancy. Conversely, other studies suggest that obese infertile women may benefit from weight loss, which may also boost self-esteem and lessen depression.[9]

IMPROVING YOUR ENVIRONMENT

Decreasing your exposure to heavy metals, toxic trace elements, cigarette smoke, and other environmental hazards known to compromise fertility should be another goal for men and women trying to conceive. Studies have found that smoking is associated with a lower-than-average number of sperm, a greater occurrence of abnormal sperm, and a decrease in sexual performance.[10] The same studies also suggest that smoking may lead to decreased fertility in women, increased frequency of menstrual abnormalities, and lowered age of spontaneous menopause. Even non-smokers who work around smokers are exposed to cadmium (a heavy metal) in secondhand cigarette smoke and may experience the ill effects that smokers experience. Remember that just because so-and-so smokes and *she* got pregnant doesn't mean it's okay to do so. After all, George Burns smoked, drank, and lived to a ripe old age, but many people die from those habits. A lot of variation among people falls under the heading of individual risk and genetics. Just because your brother or sister may get away with some unhealthy habit doesn't mean that you will; even related people are genetically unique.

Certain careers can lead to problems, too. Working with solvents or heavy metals like lead, mercury, or cadmium can hinder fertility. A career in the printing industry or some manufacturing settings can expose one to chemicals that decrease fertility. Pesticides and exogenous estrogens (estrogens produced from sources outside the body) are other culprits you'll read more about in the pages to come.

Polychlorinated biphenyls, or PCBs, are an environmental hazard potentially linked to deteriorating sperm quantity and quality.[11] Research shows that PCBs

A Success Story
Contributed by Katherine Zieman, N.D.

One of my patients was a young woman in her late twenties with a history of three conceptions but early miscarriages. She had been to an infertility clinic where they established that she had normal hormone levels. She came to me seeking alternative advice. She was a compulsive athlete, in the gym five to seven days a week, and ran several miles a day. Her physique was very thin, muscular, and pale—lacking in vitality. Her diet as a vegan was very clean. Her food choices were good and her sources organic, but her diet lacked protein and essential fatty acids. She altered her diet to include more protein and essential fatty acids. She also changed her exercise schedule to keep her fit but not wear her out. I also had her take essential fatty acid supplements as well as extra vitamins A and E. Herbal medicines were added that promote good uterine lining and support pregnancy. She was also given adrenal support. Over six months her health and vitality improved. After eight months she conceived again and carried a child to term.

might also have a negative effect on female fertility.[12] One of the main ways we're exposed to PCBs is through contaminated fish, so not eating the types of fish most likely to be affected is best. After reading this book, you'll know how to avoid environmental contaminants that might decrease your odds of conceiving.

ADOPTING HEALTHY HABITS

Many lifestyle factors that affect fertility are under your control. We know that exercising moderately—but not excessively—is conducive to fertility. For men, wearing tight briefs is not recommended because it increases scrotal temperature above normal and may hinder sperm health. (Whether or not this truly affects sperm is debatable, but why not err on the side of caution?) Severe stress tends to put the kibosh on fertility, so learning to relax or meditate is probably beneficial. Something as simple as avoiding commercial lubricants proven to severely inhibit sperm motility might help you on your path to parenthood.[13] In Chapter 2, we'll explore these lifestyle variables in more detail to help you make the best choices.

NATURAL MEDICINE IS ON YOUR SIDE

Infertility is an age-old problem, and long before expensive, high-tech procedures and fertility drugs were available, practitioners of natural medicine found effective solutions that are still in use today. CCM and TCM, botanical medicine, and homeopathy solve infertility problems with herbal preparations, acupuncture, and other noninvasive treatments. You'll read more about the philosophy of TCM and its use in treating male and female infertility in Chapter 10, but let's take a look at a few examples of this ancient system's ability to improve fertility.

One encouraging example of TCM's potential benefits to infertile men is illustrated by a research study published in the *Journal of Traditional Chinese Medicine* in 1997.[14] Two hundred and ninety-seven sterile men were treated with a combination of acupuncture, Chinese herbal remedies, and an injection of pilose antler essence. Almost half (47.8 percent) of the 297 men were considered "cured," and the treatment was deemed "markedly effective" for nearly 30 percent and "effective" for almost 18 percent. Treatment was only declared "ineffective" for about 7 percent of the men. In another study published in the same journal in 1990, Ju Jing Powder (a TCM formula) was effective in treating 85.4 percent of seminal abnormalities among eighty-two infertile male subjects.[15] Sperm density in semen, total number of sperm in a single ejaculation, and sperm activity rate all improved significantly.

TCM has an impressive ability to help some infertile women, too. In a study of sixty cases of infertility due to defects in the luteal phase of a woman's menstrual cycle (after ovulation), herbs to tonify the kidney and regulate the menstrual cycle were given to the women.[16] A whopping 56 percent of thirty-two uncomplicated cases resulted in pregnancy.

Botanical medicine uses the medicinal power of plants to improve health. Its track record is impressive for treating infertility. One example is *Panax ginseng* extract, which has been shown to increase the number of sperm, improve sperm movement, and increase testosterone and other hormone levels in men with fertility problems.[17] In Chapter 9, you'll learn more about the history and research behind specific herbs used to boost fertility in both men and women trying to conceive.

In Chapter 11 you'll read about homeopathy, a safe, time-tested system operating on the principle of "like cures like." We'll also explain how to find a skilled practitioner to help you use these forms of natural medicine.

INCREASING YOUR ODDS

Improving your health in hopes of conceiving and bringing to term a healthy, happy baby may increase your odds of doing just that. The purpose of maximizing fertility is to optimize both partners' overall health to create the most fertile, positive environment possible for conception and the resulting pregnancy to occur. The research that supports enhancing fertility naturally by nourishing the body from conception throughout the birth of a healthy baby is compelling, and taking the time to become educated about it is vitally important. When it comes to the process of nurturing a healthy baby, the old adage that input equals output most definitely applies.

It takes two to get pregnant the old-fashioned way. When both people in a couple make a concerted effort and investment in trying to do so, it becomes a bonding experience. As each person invests in his or her overall health while working to create a more fertile ground for pregnancy, their efforts are fruitful at multiple levels. As in a business acquisition, the goal is not only a net profit, but also dividends—a higher quality of life for you and your partner.

2

Improving Your Health for Enhanced Fertility

nhancing fertility is just one of the reasons that men and women hoping to conceive should focus on optimizing their health. Another motivation is that if both parents are well nourished—mentally and physically—being pregnant can be a more enjoyable experience. When the baby does arrive, healthy parents are more likely to be fit, on the ball, and ready to care for a totally dependent little one.

Making the most of your health involves tending to the well-being of your mind and your relationship, exercising, and taking care of your body by eating nutrient-rich foods, taking supplements, and avoiding dietary and environmental hazards that may hinder fertility. Of course, being as healthy as you can be doesn't guarantee you'll conceive, but it may improve your odds. In this chapter, we'll guide you through the process of making the most of your health. After some basic recommendations, we'll outline specific suggestions for men and women.

THE IMPORTANCE OF A HEALTHY RELATIONSHIP

It's important to feel confident that you and your partner have a strong, solid, trusting relationship as you think about becoming parents. In addition to general relationship issues, make time to discuss issues surrounding the potential new addition to your family. For example, what does having a baby mean to each of you? Where will the birthing process take place and who will be involved? It's also a good idea to consider questions about religion, education, in-laws, lifestyle priorities, and names before you embark on the journey toward parenthood.

One aspect of optimizing health is reducing stress in your life. Feeling prepared for the arrival of a baby as you try to conceive can help put your mind at ease. Are the relationship and family prepared for the new addition? What changes need to be made, if any? Is the house safe for a new arrival?

Parenthood also brings financial responsibility. Even child-free relationships can crumble around financial stresses. Being proactive and budgeting ahead is crucial to easing stress and maintaining your mental health as you attempt to conceive. The aim is to increase your enjoyment of the path to parenthood. When you factor in the cost of diapers, baby food, clothes, medical bills, and other costs of having a baby—as well as sleep deprivation from nighttime feedings and changes in your life's structure—you can be overwhelmed if you're not prepared.

As with any other major decision in life, thinking the process through ahead of time and being very clear about what each partner really feels, believes, and expects is absolutely critical. If someone were to buy a house without discussing the pros and cons of every location and option with his or her partner, the silent partner could become disenchanted over time. It's possible to move from a house, but having a child and signing on for raising a child are lifelong commitments well worth serious discussion ahead of time.

STRIKING A BALANCE

Another aspect of having a baby is finding personal balance in one's life. This might involve making lifestyle changes, either temporarily or permanently, that are con-

Homework

Here are a few questions couples should answer before conceiving:

✿ Who would be involved in the birthing process?

✿ Where would the birth take place—at home or in a hospital?

✿ What does having a baby really mean to each partner?

✿ Would the child be named after a parent or relative?

✿ Will you opt for day care or will one parent stay at home?

✿ What role, if any, would religion play in the child's upbringing?

✿ Would the child attend public or private school?

EXERCISE

Do you and your partner have the same ideas about raising a child? Try this exercise to compare your visions of child rearing: Sit down for at least fifteen minutes in a quiet place and make individual lists of how you envision raising a child. Then compare notes with your partner, discussing any differences and elaborating on your ideas.

A Success Story

Contributed by Katherine Zieman, N.D.

A longtime patient of mine, a woman in her late thirties with a five-year-old, was trying hard to conceive again. She had been unsuccessful for over two years. She was overworked as she tried to run two successful businesses as a medical professional and had no time to take care of herself; she had run herself ragged. We talked about what it takes physically to be able to conceive and about stress levels and how continued stress affects hormones and fertility. She agreed that she felt exhausted and depleted and that it would be hard to get pregnant in that state. I prescribed a homeopathic remedy specifically for depletion, fatigue, and inability to conceive. She was also given herbs and supplements for adrenal fatigue. She took it upon herself to alter her lifestyle and put herself on vacation in the middle of her cycle during ovulation to better facilitate conception. She conceived and carried a baby to full-term, while staying on the adrenal support as she continued to work full-time.

ducive to raising a child. This means avoiding potentially dangerous pastimes—everything from climbing mountains without adequate safety equipment to drag racing down mountain roads—and getting used to the idea of not going out as much at night after the little one has arrived. The transition from couple to couple-with-child equals the creation of a family. A healthy body includes a healthy mind and spirit. Minimizing stressors that could detract from optimal wellness and enjoyment of the process of having and raising a child, if addressed early, can multiply the joy of the experience.

Consider the things you currently do, and ask yourself which ones are absolute musts, that can't be cut out of your life, and which ones are nice but not necessary for long-term happiness, or ones that could occur less frequently. Talk to friends with children to find out how having children has changed their lives and what adjustments they've had to make. Both partners may have to make concessions for the good of the family, but if one partner feels like they're giving up more than the other, without mutual agreement on who will give up what, problems can arise. Clear communication is always best, especially if it can prevent conflicts before they arise.

Homework

1. Each partner should make a list of activities
he or she does that are musts, as well as a list of
those that are not necessary for long-term happiness, or
that could occur less often. Some examples of things that are
probably best to get rid of include going to dance clubs and staying
out most of the night, sleeping in until noon and taking naps whenever
you want, or activities that would land you on daytime talk shows. The
kinds of activities to keep in your life include hobbies, recreational reading, singing groups, and so on—things that sustain your inner energy
and interest in life. Having kids doesn't mean you won't have a life; it
just means that you have to find a balance between being responsible
for your own well-being and being there for your children who will look to
you for security and safety and as a role model. Next, compare notes
and decide together what kinds of compromises are feasible for each
partner for the overall health and happiness of a family.

2. Each partner should interview two to three people of the same gender
who have children, asking the following questions, then comparing
notes:

   ✿ How has your life changed since having a child/children?

   ✿ What adjustments have you had to make?

   ✿ What personal compromises did you make to allow for time to enjoy
   the evolution of your family?

3. Each partner should answer the following questions, then compare
answers:

   ✿ Is one partner willing to give up his or her career to stay at home
   with the child (if that makes sense financially)?

   ✿ Are there things that one or both partners are absolutely opposed
   to giving up?

   ✿ Does having a family still make sense, considering the factors
   discussed?

CREATING A HEALTHY ENVIRONMENT

Think about the kind of environment to which you want to expose a child. Granted, there are many factors beyond your control, but do the best you can to adopt a lifestyle relative to your habits, friends, and the kind of environment you want for a child.

Consider if your current lifestyle allows enough time for the addition of a little one. As a parent-to-be, do you allow for time to stay grounded and balanced, or are you uptight, stressed out, and easily irritated? If you smoke in the house, do you want your baby to be exposed to secondhand smoke or its chemicals on clothing, furniture, bedding, or in the air? Would you be willing to give up smoking for the health of your child and for your own well-being? If you use illegal drugs, are you ready to stop?

Working on these issues prior to the arrival of your baby is important. It will make the experience of parenthood that much more sweet, enjoyable, and rewarding. Remember: A baby is like a sponge in the sense that he or she soaks up and imprints what he or she is exposed to, whether it's positive or negative. You make a decision about your actions and the baby lives with it, adapting to the best of its little ability.

Would you want your children to adopt your current lifestyle, habits, and risks, or would you want your kids to see what you are doing? The reality is that parents are the role models for their offspring. Your children will one day be in the exact position you're in right now: preparing for the next generation of your family tree. Making sure that the roots of that tree are healthy enough to support strong and sturdy branches will ensure that the family will be able to weather the storms of life together and that branches will not be lost along the way.

Since your baby—then toddler, child, teenager—will count on both parents for years to come, taking good care of yourself now is essential. After working so hard to have a baby, it only makes sense that you would want to live to see your kids and grandkids grow up and succeed. You need good health to be there for your kids and for yourself—and to spoil your future grandchildren. Do your best to ensure that you will have the best quality of life possible.

One can be old chronologically, but who wants to feel his or her age? There is a difference between biological age (health age) and chronological age (actual years). A person who is seventy years old may have a biological age of fifty or eighty-plus years, depending on their genetics and how well they've taken care of themselves. We all know people many years older than we are who can run circles around us.

There is a saying that genetics loads the gun, yet lifestyle and diet pull the trigger. You can't change your genetic makeup, but you can make the most of it by taking good care of yourself. Investing in your health early on is like putting money in the bank; it collects interest over time and can pay big dividends.

FOCUS ON A HEALTHY DIET

Eating a balanced, healthy diet is necessary for your body to function properly, and has proven to decrease the risk of diseases like cancer and heart disease. Eating right may also improve your odds of conceiving and giving birth to a healthy baby. Deficiencies of some nutrients, which we'll discuss below, are thought to decrease fertility. Not everyone agrees on exactly what constitutes a healthy diet, but basic tenets of healthy eating founded on solid scientific research are virtually irrefutable.

Eating the Right Amount of Food

One dietary concern related to fertility is simply that you are eating the right amount of food. Eating disorders including anorexia nervosa and bulimia nervosa in women can hinder fertility, as well as negatively affect menstruation, maternal weight gain, fetal well-being, and overall health. Roughly 12 percent of cases of primary infertility (infertility without any previous pregnancy) that are caused by problems with ovulation are linked to abnormal weight. Weighing 85 percent or less of ideal weight was linked in one study to a nearly five-fold increase in infertility risk related to ovulation. Likewise, risk of infertility was doubled in subjects weighing 120 percent or more of ideal weight.[1] Catherine Downey, N.D., Associate Dean of Clinical and Graduate Medical Education at the National College of Naturopathic Medicine in Portland, Oregon, recommends that thin female patients gain 5 to 10 pounds to increase their odds of conceiving. She notes that weighing less than 85 percent of a woman's ideal weight decreases the likelihood of conception by three to four times.

Severe reducing diets cause low levels of the hormone progesterone, a female sex hormone made by the ovaries that helps prepare the endometrium (uterus lining) for implantation of a fertilized egg. Progesterone also prepares the mammary glands to secrete milk. Severe reducing diets can also slow follicle growth, inhibit the surge of luteinizing hormone (LH) needed around ovulation, and prevent ovulation from occurring. Even less severe slimming can depress hormone levels by producing a corpus luteum that is too small, which may result in miscarriage. The corpus luteum is an endocrine gland in the ovary that is formed after a follicle discharges its secondary oocyte (the form of the egg released at ovulation). The gland secretes estrogens, progesterone, and other important hormones crucial to healthy reproductive function.

In a study published in the *American Journal of Obstetrics and Gynecology,* 7.6 percent of women in an infertility clinic were found to suffer from anorexia nervosa or bulimia nervosa.[2] When eating disorders not otherwise specified were included, researchers found that a total of 16.7 percent of infertility patients in the study suffered from eating disorders. Another study, published in the *Journal of Clinical Psychiatry,* reported that women with anorexia nervosa had significantly more miscarriages and caesarean deliveries.[3] Offspring of women with anorexia were more likely to be born prematurely and weigh less at birth than offspring of non-anorexic women. Babies born to anorexic women with no history of bulimia nervosa had lower body weight than those born to anorexic women with a lifetime history of bulimia nervosa. The researchers found no difference between women with active versus remitted anorexia nervosa on any of the measures in the study.

The relationship between eating disorders and decreased reproductive success is one of nature's protective measures. When food intake is inadequate, the body suspends reproductive attempts in favor of processes crucial for survival of the individual. After all, if a woman does not survive, her unborn baby can't. If the woman does survive, there is a chance that she may get pregnant later, when nutrient intake is high enough to support both mother and child.

We know that farmland with depleted soil is less likely to nourish a seed. Land that is depleted, then flooded by a local river, often becomes abundantly fertile. Likewise, bathing the body in nutrients replenishes the critical building blocks for the parent's body, thus creating optimally fertile ground.

Many women with a history of eating disorders do have the ability to get pregnant and give birth to healthy babies, and many do just that. A study published in the *American Journal of Psychiatry* in 2002 found that, while menstrual irregularities are common in women who have bulimia nervosa, the disorder appears to have little effect on a woman's ability to achieve pregnancy later.[4] One of many success stories is a report in a nursing journal about a twenty-six-year-old woman who battled anorexia and bulimia ten years prior, then became pregnant, delivered a healthy infant at term, and was successfully breast-feeding it at five months.[5]

The studies cited above illustrate the importance of both eating enough nutritious food and having a healthy relationship with food, which your body absolutely needs to nourish you and a fetus. Evidence suggests that the minimum ratio of fat to lean mass typically needed by women to menstruate is 17 percent of body weight as fat.[6] To maintain reproductive ability, evidence shows that women need, at the minimum, approximately 22 percent of body weight as fat. This helps maintain regularity of cycles and ovulation patterns.

Women with eating disorders often appear to have normal weight and may not inform their doctors of their condition. If you have or have had an eating disorder, be sure to tell your doctor so that he or she will know your history. Intensive prenatal care for women with both active and remitted anorexia nervosa is especially important to ensure good prenatal nutrition and fetal development. Knowing your history, your doctor can help you adopt a healthier way of eating to nourish yourself and—if all goes well—a growing fetus. A knowledgeable practitioner may be able to give you a recovery diet designed for people trying to overcome eating disorders.

At the other end of the scale, being overweight or obese compromises one's health, too, increasing the risk of diseases and other health problems. If this is a concern, talk to your doctor about how you might achieve a healthier weight through diet and lifestyle modifications. Body Mass Index, or BMI, which was established by the National Institutes of Health in 1998, is a better indicator than the bathroom scale for estimating body fat and the health risks associated with being overweight or underweight. You can calculate your BMI by entering your height and weight measurements into the BMI formula. A BMI between 18.5 and 24 is considered the most desirable, a BMI between 25 and 30 is considered overweight, and a BMI of 30 or more is considered obese. To learn more about BMI, visit the Mayo Clinic website at www.MayoClinic.com and search for BMI.

Homework

CALCULATE YOUR BODY MASS INDEX (BMI)

1. (Your weight in pounds) x 0.45 = X
2. (Your height in inches) x 0.025 = Y
3. Then take X divided by (Y x Y) = BMI

   18.5 to 24: most desirable

   25 to 30: overweight

   30 or more: obese

If your BMI suggests that you are underweight, overweight, or obese, talk to your doctor about striving toward a healthier weight through lifestyle modifications. Your practitioner should be able to help you reach and maintain a healthy weight. It is worth noting, however, that studies suggest that a woman should not lose a *lot* of weight right before getting pregnant. If she does, she should wait, ideally, six months before trying to get pregnant. The rationale behind this is that toxins stored in fat tissues are released with weight loss, and they should have a chance to leave the body. Though this waiting period is ideal, a woman shouldn't worry about it if she does get pregnant sooner.

Because there is so much individual variation among people, there's no magic number of calories that can be recommended per day. Somebody who is very active is going to need more calories than someone who is sedentary, and variation in body size and metabolic rate also affect a person's caloric needs. Don't get caught up on counting calories. Instead, listen to your body's cues about how much to eat. Eat slowly and stop when you're full. Sit down at the table, turn off the television, and focus on your food instead of eating on the run or when you're distracted. This will help you actually enjoy your meals and enable you to hear your body cuing you that you've had enough. Eating the right foods is another large piece of the healthy pie. Also, bear in mind that overexercising can still cause a caloric and nutrient deficit. If you are wondering whether you are overexercising, ask your healthcare provider.

Choosing the Best Diet: Plentiful Plant Foods

A person doesn't have to be anorexic or bulimic to be malnourished. Living on refined carbohydrates, cookies, candy, pasta, bread, and noodles, and not eating enough vegetables, fruit, and protein can cause deficiencies regardless of the amount of calories consumed. What foods should you be eating?

For starters, it would be difficult to overstate the importance of fresh fruits and vegetables in a healthy diet. The U.S. Department of Agriculture (USDA) recommends two to four servings of fruit per day and three to five servings of vegetables per day for good reason. These foods contain calories, fiber, carbohydrates, vitamins, minerals, and other beneficial components (like antioxidants) that we all need for everyday functions, as well as for growth, energy, disease prevention, and more.

An impressive body of scientific evidence has found that a diet rich in plant foods protects against many diseases common in Western society and that a low intake of plant foods contributes to disease development. Besides fruits and vegetables, eating plentiful plant foods like whole grains and legumes benefits health and decreases disease risk. It has also been estimated that one-third of cancers are related to diet. Low intake of dietary fiber, low fruit and vegetable consumption, and high red-meat consumption are associated with colon and other kinds of cancer, and experts agree that diet may affect cancer development.

Organic produce is best, so choose it over commercial produce, if you can afford it. Otherwise, plant a garden or join a community food co-op to avoid pesticides and other contaminants that commercial produce may contain.

Up the Antioxidants

Fruits and vegetables are high in antioxidants, which protect the body from damage by free radicals. Free radicals are highly reactive molecules that come from environmental toxins (such as cigarette smoke), and some are even produced in the body as byproducts of normal metabolism. Free radicals contain an unpaired electron, making them chemically unstable; they steal electrons from stable molecules in order to stabilize themselves and thereby create more free radicals. They damage cells and even DNA (your body's genetic material) in the process. Eating a lot of fried or chemical-laden foods and drinking too much alcohol can harm chromosomes due to free-radical damage, which contributes to aging, heart disease, cancer, and other serious health problems.

DNA damage, including that from free radicals, can have a negative impact on reproduction, as well. DNA is passed down from each parent to offspring via chromosomes. Each parent contributes twenty-three chromosomes to the baby in the sperm and the egg. This genetic material carries the mapping that is unique to each parent—eye and hair color, genetic tendencies, and other characteristics. The genetic material is somewhat analogous to a bar code on a product at the supermarket; keeping the lines in order is important so that the right message is communicated. For example, if you had a carton of milk and moved around the little bars in the bar code, the scan might identify it as a box of cereal instead. Likewise, if your DNA is damaged, it may lead to abnormalities in the developing fetus. For example, instead of four fingers and a thumb the result could be six digits. This kind of miscommunication can also cause Down syndrome, a disorder resulting from an error in cell division that causes mental retardation and problems with physical development and malformation. Unhealthy maternal habits such as smoking and drinking alcohol may increase the risk of having a baby with Down syndrome because these habits are known to alter genetic material. When the mixing of genetic material from both parents occurs, you do not want to have something like a free-radical-driven tornado that prevents the properly ordered mixing of chromosomes.

What's wonderful about antioxidants is that they protect us from free-radical damage by quenching those harmful molecules—by donating electrons to stabilize them—while remaining relatively stable themselves. When we eat fruits, vegetables, and other foods high in antioxidants, we protect ourselves, to some degree, from free-radical damage. Some examples of antioxidants are vitamins E and C, lycopene, and beta-carotene, among many others. In this chapter, as well as in later chapters, we'll talk more about how much of these nutrients you should be getting from foods and supplements on a daily basis. The emphasis here is on eating plenty of fresh fruits and vegetables (again, organic are best), which will provide you with many beneficial antioxidants and other invaluable nutrients.

It helps to remember that living in today's environment is very challenging, and all you can ever do is your best, based on what you know at any given time. So many people make unintentional mistakes regarding their health. From this point on, you and your partner should be better informed, armed with knowledge that many, if not most, of your friends and family don't yet have. You may even be able to help someone else by sharing what you learn in these pages.

More Nutritious News

Drink up—water, that is. Drink at least six to eight 8-ounce glasses of filtered water every day. Try to avoid tap water, unless you know it does not contain chlorine, heavy metals (like lead from old pipes), or contaminants from unpure water sources. Often a reasonably priced carbon-based filter that will decrease exposure to potentially harmful substances can be attached to your faucet without special tools. Be sure to read the filter's label to see what it removes from the water. That way, you can choose a filter with the best protection. You'll read more about water filters later in this chapter.

Research about the effects of caffeine (from coffee and other sources) on fertility has turned up conflicting results, but it's probably best for both men and women who are trying to conceive to err on the side of caution and drastically reduce, if not eliminate, caffeine from the diet. Observational studies suggest that caffeine reduces fertility, at least in women. We know caffeine reduces prolactin concentration in the blood, and low levels are associated with infertility in females.[7] There's not much evidence that caffeine affects male fertility but, again, it may be wise to limit intake, just in case. Catherine Downey, N.D., advises her female patients to avoid caffeine, smoking, and alcohol.

Alcohol may negatively affect sperm health in men and fertility in women, so abstaining from drinking when trying to conceive is a good idea. Even drinking moderate amounts of alcohol might contribute to infertility in women,[8] because alcohol is known to deplete nutrients. While hard liquor should be avoided, an occasional glass of wine may be harmless but, again, abstinence is best. Even moderate alcohol consumption, Downey cautions, may decrease conception for a given cycle.

If you do eat meat, minimize your consumption of red meat and poultry that has been commercially raised. Hormones and antibiotics are often used in raising commercial livestock in the United States, leaving the long-term and potentially harmful effects on offspring uncertain. The concentration of environmental toxins (such as pesticides) in a given food tends to correlate to its place on the food chain: the higher up the food chain, the higher the concentration of toxins. So there will likely be higher concentrations of these toxic compounds in animal flesh or dairy products than in plant foods. If you choose to eat meat and dairy, seek out organic or free-range varieties, which have become more readily available. Following these guidelines is wise, but becoming *too* zealous about what you eat can also increase your stress and potentially have a negative effect on your health. The key to a healthy life is moderation and stress management.

Fat Facts

There's a lot of confusion about fat in the diet these days, and it's no wonder. It's a complex topic, and research results are sometimes conflicting. Even so, there are some things we do know about fat that can help us improve our diet and optimize our health.

Banish Bad Fats

Here are some fats to avoid as you strive for optimal health:

✿ Saturated fats: animal fats, coconut and palm oils

✿ Trans-fatty acids: partially hydrogenated oils found in most processed foods, such as chips, crackers, and cookies

✿ Cottonseed oil: contains gossypol, a substance that may decrease sperm function

Four major kinds of fats are found in foods we eat: cholesterol, monounsaturated fat, poly-unsaturated fat, and saturated fat. Though too much cholesterol can be bad for health, small amounts are actually needed for hormone production and other functions. Omega-9 oleic acid is the main monounsaturated fatty acid (MUFA) in foods such as olives (and olive oil) and avocados. Omega-3 and omega-6 fatty acids are the major types of polyunsaturated fats (PUFAs) found in foods. Both classes of PUFAs (omega-3s and omega-6s) are considered essential fatty acids because we must get them from the diet; the body cannot manufacture them.

Dietary sources of omega-6s include safflower, corn, and sunflower oil, whereas the main source of omega-3 fatty acids is fish. The ratio of omega-6 to omega-3 fatty acid intake is currently about 10:1 or higher among people in the United States. This is partly because Americans eat relatively little fish. Many researchers consider a 4:1 ratio of omega-6 to omega-3 fatty acids a good goal. Clearly, most of us get plenty of omega-6s in our diets, but not enough omega-3s.

The omega-3 class of PUFAs includes three forms you should remember. *Alpha-linolenic acid,* or ALA, is not found in many foods. Some seed oils, walnuts, and leafy greens do contain ALA, with flax oil being a very rich source. The body converts ALA to *eicosapentaenoic acid* (EPA), another omega-3 fatty acid with important physiological roles. EPA, along with *docosahexaenoic acid* (DHA, another omega-3 fatty acid), is also found in cold-water fish oils.

While the body, according to some research, may not be able to convert ALA to the longer-chain DHA and EPA very efficiently, some practitioners believe that ALA sources such as flaxseed oil are sufficient to meet the body's omega-3 needs.

For example, Katherine Zieman, N.D., a naturopathic doctor and midwife who also counsels infertile couples, recommends evening primrose oil as a good source of EFAs, although it is more expensive than flaxseed oil. Think of it as an investment in your health.

Saturated fat, found primarily in animal products, is associated with increased risk of heart disease, so limiting foods high in this kind of fat is best. Trans-fatty acids, which have been linked to an increased risk of heart disease, should also be avoided as much as possible. Trans-fatty acids are found in margarine, shortening, and products containing partially hydrogenated vegetable oils, such as packaged cookies and crackers. Cottonseed oil, which is used occasionally in processed foods and medicinal preparations, should be limited or avoided, ideally, due to its potential negative effect on male fertility.

Have a Healthy Heart

Our bodies need EFAs for many functions, including production of hormones.

Homework

Do some detective work in your pantry and refrigerator to eradicate fats that might compromise your health.

1. Take out all the boxes of crackers, cookies, and other processed snacks and foods, lining them up on your kitchen counter.

2. One by one, read the ingredient lists and set aside those that contain partially hydrogenated oils, cottonseed oil, coconut and palm oils, and animal fats. (You may be surprised how pervasive they are.)

3. Decide which of those products you are willing to throw away. If it's not economically feasible to do so now, make a list of products that you won't buy next time, based on their unsavory ingredients.

4. Visit your local health food store or health food section of your grocery store and seek out healthier alternatives free of these fats (raw almonds or crisp breads free of hydrogenated oils instead of crackers, for example). In doing so, you'll likely cut nonnutritive additives and preservatives from your diet, as well.

EFAs are also necessary for the health of sperm cell membranes; a deficiency leads to faulty formation of cell membranes. DHA is a crucial part of cellular membranes, especially in the brain and retina of the eye. It is essential to the growth and development of infant brains and is needed to maintain normal brain function in adults, too. But one of the most critical roles of EFAs is reducing the risk of heart disease, which kills roughly half a million Americans—men and women—each year. Omega-3 fatty acids keep inflammatory processes associated with coronary artery disease in check.

If our intake of omega-6s isn't balanced by omega-3s, an omega-6 called arachidonic acid can actually encourage heart attack, atherosclerosis, and fatal cardiac arrhythmias. Inflammation caused by arachidonic acid plays a major role in promoting the development and buildup of plaques in coronary arteries; continuing damage by inflammation can eventually lead to narrowing or entire blockage of the coronary artery, resulting in a heart attack. Arachidonic acid also increases platelet aggregation (or stickiness), potentially causing blood clots that, when large enough, can block blood flow and result in a heart attack. Animal flesh is high in arachidonic acid. The omega 3s EPA and DHA, conversely, reduce platelet stickiness and clotting, also preventing plaque buildup by raising levels of HDL, the "good" cholesterol. There is also evidence that omega-3s may lower levels of LDL, sometimes called the "bad" cholesterol. The actions of both omega-3s and omega-6s are largely due to their role in creating prostaglandins in the body, which affect constriction and dilation of blood vessels and blood clotting. Omega-3 fatty acids increase blood flow to and from the heart by relaxing and dilating blood vessels. They reduce the risk of sudden cardiac death, too. Many people who die right away after a heart attack experience cardiac arrhythmias—erratic electrical activity of heart cells that hinders the heart's pumping action, halting blood flow to organs including the brain. Omega-3s help reduce abnormal electrical activity, providing the body with protection against arrhythmias. For an illustration of omega-3 and omega-6 pathways, please see Figure 2.1. As shown in the figure, key nutrients must also be present in one's diet to gain the full benefit from EFAs.

In summary, we each have a muscle in our body, a 10-ounce heart that contracts some 110,000 times every day from before birth to the end of our lives. Taking care of this paramount pump called the heart is essential. The saying "it's all a matter of heart" can be used to sum up health. The healthy heart delivers the oxygen and nutrients that fuel trillions of cells throughout every millimeter of our bodies comprising our brains and other organs. There is no single more debilitating condition than having a heart that can't keep the body properly fueled.

OMEGA-3 PATHWAY

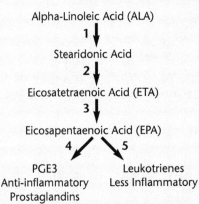

Alpha-Linoleic Acid (ALA)
1 ↓
Stearidonic Acid
2 ↓
Eicosatetraenoic Acid (ETA)
3 ↓
Eicosapentaenoic Acid (EPA)
4 ↙   ↘ 5

PGE3   Leukotrienes
Anti-inflammatory   Less Inflammatory
Prostaglandins

1. Delta-6-desaturase turns ALA into stearidonic acid. This step requires sufficient B_6, magnesium, and zinc.

2. Elongase turns stearidonic acid into ETA.

3. Delta-5-desaturase converts ETA into EPA, and requires B_3, vitamin C, and zinc.

4. Cyclo-oxygenase (COX) enzyme converts EPA into PGE3.

5. Lipoxygenase enzyme converts EPA into leukotrienes.

OMEGA-6 PATHWAY

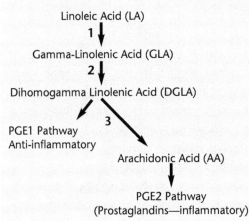

Linoleic Acid (LA)
1 ↓
Gamma-Linolenic Acid (GLA)
2 ↓
Dihomogamma Linolenic Acid (DGLA)
↙   ↘ 3
PGE1 Pathway
Anti-inflammatory

Arachidonic Acid (AA)
↓
PGE2 Pathway
(Prostaglandins—inflammatory)

1. Delta-6-desaturase converts LA into GLA (requires B_6, magnesium, and zinc).

2. Elongase turns GLA into DGLA.

3. Delta-5-desaturase converts DGLA to AA (requires B_3, Vitamin C, and zinc).

FIGURE 2.1. EFA Pathways

Every aspect of your health is dependent upon having enough of the right building blocks from food so that that the biochemical pathways in your body are properly fueled. A perfect illustration of your body's dependence on the right nutrients at the right time is essential fatty acid pathways within your body. Essential fatty acids, by definition, must be consumed in the form of food or supplements, yet for them to perform their intended function within your body, they need the right vitamins and minerals present.

EFA pathways require sufficient magnesium, zinc, vitamin B_3, vitamin B_6, and vitamin C. Deficiency in any of these nutrients can lead to inflammation, aches and pains, asthma, and problems with cholesterol and cellular function.

Seeking Out Sources of EFAs

Much of the research on omega-3s has been done with fish and fish oil, which contain EPA and DHA. Eating fish is one way to get more of both these omega-3s. Just be sure to limit your intake of tuna and other fish more likely to be contaminated with mercury or cancer-causing pollutants such as PCBs, especially if there's a chance you could be pregnant. Freshwater fish are more likely to be contaminated than ocean species. Healthy alternatives include migratory Atlantic or Pacific salmon, deep-water halibut, and Atlantic cod.

The source of fish that you eat is critical. When sewage is dumped into or spills into a local river, residents are warned not to swim or eat fish from that water for a period of time. The reality, however, is that once fish consume something, it is incorporated into their tissues (what we call "fillets"). It's great to have tasty fish, but the flavor should be a result of the cooking process and not what the fish swam in. Not a very mouth-watering thought, is it?

If you want a supplement to increase your intake of EFAs, seek out a fish-oil supplement highly concentrated in EPA and DHA (at least 50 percent omega-3 content, preferably higher). Many products have less omega-3s and more omega-9s, omega-6s, and other lipids; these are considered less desirable. Read labels for recommended dosages. Antioxidant vitamins C and E taken with these supplements protect the omega-3s from oxidation. People taking blood thinners including warfarin or aspirin, as well as women who are pregnant or lactating, should consult their healthcare provider before taking any omega-3 supplements.

Controversy continues about the body's ability to convert ALA to DHA and EPA, yet vegetarians or people wary of eating any fish products due to potential contamination are better off eating foods high in ALA—flaxseed, purslane, walnut, perilla, and other land-based plants. Choose organic, cold expeller–pressed brands of flaxseed oil, which is a highly concentrated source of ALA, from your health food store refrigerator. Chase the liquid flaxseed oil with juice or another beverage if the taste is unappealing. It can also be drizzled on salads, and the seeds can be ground up with a coffee grinder and sprinkled on cereal, vegetables, or yogurt. Flaxseed oil is relatively inexpensive in liquid form and is also available in capsules. These oils, whether in liquid or capsule form, are unstable and should be refrigerated in tinted, airtight containers. Don't use them for cooking and throw them away if they smell rancid. For cooking and other applications, olive oil is a good choice.

Chew on This

Consider boosting your intake of these nutrient-dense foods to optimize your health. Many of them make good snacks, too.

- **Fresh, organic fruits and vegetables.** Add fresh color to your plate for better health; opt for more greens (kale, bok choy, and various lettuce varieties), red cabbage, blueberries, cherries, and other colorful fruits and vegetables. Cooked tomato products eaten with a fat source (olive oil in pasta sauce, for example) are the best sources of lycopene, a potent antioxidant linked to prostate and overall health. Aim for a colorful salad a day and have a bowl of fresh fruit for snacking. Steam or lightly sauté vegetables instead of frying them.

- **Almonds, walnuts, and other raw, unsalted nuts.** Grab a small handful of nuts for a nutritious snack, or add chopped nuts to salads and other dishes. Nuts add flavor and nutritional value when they are added to baked goods, such as low-fat muffins and breads.

- **Pumpkin, sunflower, and sesame seeds.** Eat these in dried or roasted form, alone or sprinkled in salads.

- **Cold-processed flaxseed oil, evening primrose oil, and flaxseeds.** These can be mixed with fresh herbs and drizzled on salads and other foods or added to smoothies. Adding flaxseeds to the diet increases the length of a woman's luteal phase (the phase following ovulation), her luteal phase progesterone/estrogen ratio, and her mid-follicular testosterone concentration—all of which promote conception, according to Catherine Downey, N.D.

- **Legumes.** Beans are high in fiber, protein, and other beneficial components. Consider cooking soups that include beans, or add some beans to your favorite salads for a hearty nutrient boost. Soybeans and soy products (such as tofu, meat analogs, and soy protein powder for use in smoothies) are widely available and, in small amounts can be good additions to the diet. Soybeans contain isoflavones, which are phytoestrogens, or plant compounds that weakly mimic the action of estrogen in the body. Isoflavones are beneficial to health, but it may be best to limit consumption of isoflavones to amounts typical of diets in cultures where soy is consumed regularly (Japan, for instance) to avoid possible changes in the body's hormones. (People in Asian countries haven't traditionally consumed a lot of concentrated soy products as many Americans now do.) If you are having trouble conceiving and you eat soy foods regularly, ask your doctor if you should decrease your intake and substitue other lean protein sources such as nuts and seeds and organic, low-fat dairy products. Too many isoflavones may increase the length of the follicular phase of the menstrual cycle and delay ovulation, notes Downey.

- **Whole wheat, brown rice, and other unrefined grains.** High in fiber and low in calories, these complex carbohydrates are excellent foods. They also contain nutrients that are lost during the refining process, making them superior to refined products. (People with celiac disease, however, can't tolerate the gluten in wheat, rye, oats, and barley.) Choose whole-grain over white bread, and steam or boil brown rice and top with steamed veggies and spices for a healthy dinner. Try cooked oatmeal with nuts, chopped fruit, and soymilk for breakfast. Polenta, or cooked cornmeal (corn is also considered a grain), can be used like pasta in recipes.

Nutrient Recommendations

Several nutrients, including some of the antioxidants discussed above, play specific roles in fertility. Here's a look at several of them. (Vitamin and mineral therapy for infertility will be covered more thoroughly in later chapters.)

VITAMIN C

In addition to protecting cells from free radicals, vitamin C is thought to be associated with fertility because it promotes collagen synthesis and aids in hormone production. Also called ascorbic acid, vitamin C is found in both the ovary and the testes, suggesting that it is important for reproduction in both men and women. Researchers believe that the cycles of tissue remodeling and peptide and steroid secretion that take place in male and female gonads depend on vitamin C.[9]

This well-known vitamin might also prevent free-radical damage to gametes (the male and female reproductive cells: the spermatozoa and ova) during production and fertilization. Depleted levels of vitamin C in females may contribute to destruction of the corpus luteum, which forms after ovulation from the mature ovarian follicle that ruptures and expels an egg.[10] The high concentration of vitamin C in semen helps maintain the genetic integrity of sperm by preventing oxidative damage to its DNA. Vitamin C supplementation has been found to enhance fertility in infertile men. You'll read more about this exciting research in Chapter 8, which focuses on nutritional medicine.

Animal studies have also demonstrated that dietary supplementation with a mix of vitamins C and E may prevent a decrease in the ovulation rate in older females.[11] While it's too soon to extrapolate the results to humans, it does suggest that supplementation with these vitamins might help prevent or delay infertility in older women. There are plenty of other well-established reasons to make sure you're getting enough of these and other vitamins through a balanced diet and good multivitamin and mineral supplementation.

Bonus: Vitamin C supports the immune system, helping protect against viruses and bacteria.

Rich Sources: Citrus fruits, broccoli, peppers, Brussels sprouts, potatoes.

ZINC

Zinc is another nutrient of paramount importance to reproductive health, especially in men. It is involved in the production of testosterone and the formation of sperm, and low levels of zinc are associated with infertility in men. Also, low blood levels of testosterone have been associated with low zinc levels. Zinc supplementation has been shown to boost sperm count and sperm motility in men with oligospermia (scanty secretion of sperm).[12] Zinc is absolutely necessary for the health of prostate and testicular tissue.

Bonus: Zinc is needed to maintain vision, taste, and smell. An antioxidant, this mineral may scavenge free radicals in semen following ejaculation.

Rich Sources: Shellfish, fish, oysters, red meat, nuts, seeds, legumes, whole grains.

VITAMIN E

When vitamin E was discovered in 1922, it was referred to as "the fertility vitamin." That's because scientists discovered that animals deficient in vitamin E became sterile. Now we know that this antioxidant plays a number of other important protective roles in health, but its relationship with reproduction is still among its most notable attributes.

Some infertile men tend to have high levels of free radicals and low levels of antioxidants in their semen. Vitamin E protects sperm from lipid peroxidation (free-radical damage to fats) in the cell membrane. This damage impairs sperm motility, a condition called *asthenospermia*. Boosting vitamin E in the diet and with supplementation can help keep sperm healthy. In one study, subjects with asthenospermia taking oral vitamin E experienced decreased lipid peroxidation in sperm and improved motility.[13] Eleven of fifty-two treated patients, or 21 percent, impregnated their spouses; nine of the pregnancies resulted in normal deliveries.

Bonus: Vitamin E has also become famous for its ability to help keep the heart healthy and protect LDL, the "bad" form of cholesterol, from becoming oxidized and stickier, thereby preventing it from adhering to artery walls where it can eventually lead to blockage.

Rich Sources: Seeds, nuts, polyunsaturated vegetable oils, whole grains, avocados, tomatoes, asparagus, berries, leafy green vegetables.

ARGININE

Supplemental L-arginine, an amino acid, can improve fertility in men and women. In one recent study, it was shown to improve ovarian response to gonadotropin (a stimulant to the gonads) in women undergoing assisted reproduction who had not previously responded well.[14] It also improved other fertility-related factors among women. Arginine is especially helpful for men with sperm counts of 20 million or more (in the normal range), but it may also be worth including in the health plan for men with lower counts. Supplementation with arginine has been shown to improve sperm count in men with oligospermia,[15] and some research has found it to be effective in cases of asthenospermia.[16] This amino acid is essential for cell replication, including sperm formation.

Bonus: Arginine has also been shown to help with increased erectile strength and fullness due to its effect on the nitric oxide levels that cause vasodilation (dilation of blood vessels). It may have similar effects on the clitoris. (Those suffering from kidney disease, herpes, or other infections should use arginine very cautiously because it promotes cell replication and may cause a breakout.)

Rich Sources: Peanuts, soybeans, hazelnuts, shrimp, chicken breast, tuna, wheat germ.

L-CARNITINE

Carnitine, another amino acid, is necessary for normal sperm function. Once metabolized, it helps flagellar sperm movement, which is the whiplike motion of the sperm tail that propels it forward. It also has a protective effect that improves sperm survival and, hence, fertility.[17] Hypomotility, a problem of sperm movement, is thought to be due to an intrasperm L-carnitine deficiency, so taking L-carnitine or boosting its uptake may improve motility.[18] In at least one study supplementation with L-carnitine for four months increased sperm count and motility in infertile men with primary asthenospermia.[19]

Bonus: Carnitine is also important for proper heart function.

Rich Sources: Dairy products, red meat. (The body can convert the amino acid lysine into carnitine, and legumes are good sources of lysine.)

SELENIUM

Low selenium levels in the diet might be partly to blame for low selenium status in some men. Twelve selenium-containing proteins have been identified in testicular tissue, and supplemental selenium has been shown to protect sperm from oxidative damage. Among men with impaired fertility in a double-blind, clinically controlled study, selenium supplementation increased sperm motility.[20] Five men taking selenium became fathers, while none in the placebo group did.

Bonus: This antioxidant has been shown to help maintain optimal prostate health, demonstrating that natural medicines often fuel overall health while also helping to target a specific aspect of health.

Rich Sources: Brazil nuts, wheat germ, bran, whole-wheat bread, barley, oats, red Swiss chard, brown rice.

VITAMIN B$_{12}$

This vitamin is needed for cellular replication, as well as for optimum sperm motility and total sperm count. Studies have found that 1,000 micrograms of vitamin B$_{12}$ dramatically improved sperm counts.[21]

Bonus: Vitamin B$_{12}$ is important for proper nerve functioning, and can frequently become depleted in older people and among vegetarians who don't have perfectly balanced diets.

Rich Sources: Liver, kidney, eggs, meat, fish, cheese; supplements (especially for vegans).

COENZYME Q$_{10}$

This popular antioxidant, also called ubiquinone, is found in high levels in semen and is directly correlated with sperm count and motility.[22] The same study showed that a higher concentration of CoQ$_{10}$ in sperm cells helps protect sperm membranes from free-radical damage. CoQ$_{10}$ is also important for energy production, which helps promote normal sperm activity. (The exact mechanisms are not yet known, however). Patients with low fertility taking 60 milligrams a day of CoQ$_{10}$ for 103 days had significantly improved fertilization rates.[23] Doses as small as 10 milligrams per day for a few weeks may even be enough to improve sperm count and motility.

Bonus: CoQ$_{10}$ has been shown to help bolster immune function in several conditions, and it is essential to heart health. Many people who die from heart disease have low levels of CoQ$_{10}$ in their heart tissue.

Rich Sources: Salmon, sardines, mackerel, beef heart, chicken livers, pork; lesser amounts in peanuts and broccoli; supplements (especially for vegetarians).

FOLIC ACID

Folic acid—also called folate—has a lot going for it. It is necessary for DNA synthesis and, therefore, cell division. It prevents neural tube defects, urinary tract and cardiovascular defects and decreases limb deficiencies and other problems in newborns, so it's essential for pregnant women to take it. But that's not all. Multivitamin supplementation with folic acid around the time of conception improved fertility and the rate of twins in one recent double-blind, placebo-controlled Hungarian study.[24] In Hungary, this supplement is part of periconceptual (around the time of conception) care and may improve fertility rates among women having trouble conceiving. Adequate folic acid consumption encourages optimal sperm formation, as well.

Bonus: Maintaining proper folic acid levels can also help protect against abnormal pap smears; intake is sufficient if a woman's pap smear is normal. Women who take, or have taken, birth control pills should supplement with folic acid daily because oral contraceptives deplete folic acid levels in the body. Ideally, all women should take folic acid six months prior to conception. The amount of folic acid included in prenatal vitamins is intentionally higher.

Rich Sources: Whole grains, oranges, spinach, kale, chard, beet greens, broccoli, asparagus, legumes, cabbage, root vegetables.

Ensuring Adequate Nutrient Intake

Striving to get as much nutrition as possible from the diet is a worthwhile goal. But for various reasons—depleted mineral content in soil, decreased nutrients in food by the time they go from field to store to fridge to cooking to our mouths, or even imperfect eating habits—it's not always possible to get optimal amounts of all nutrients from foods. That's where supplements come in. In Chapter 8, we'll explain how to choose the best multivitamin and mineral supplements.

Eating healthfully *and* taking a well-formulated multivitamin and mineral formula is a wise combination that will help you optimize overall health and reproductive health, in particular. Even the American Medical Association, long opposed to encouraging vitamin supplements, in June 2002 began endorsing the daily use of multivitamins by all American adults, based on overwhelming evidence that doing so can decrease disease risk and improve health.

The Recommended Dietary Allowance, or RDA, for most vitamins and minerals is very conservative, and many practitioners recommend taking higher levels of these nutrients—with the help of a high-potency vitamin and mineral supplement—for optimal health. Vitamins and minerals are very safe. The only vitamins that might cause toxicity problems at high levels in healthy people are vitamins A (pregnant women, or those hoping to become pregnant, shouldn't take more than 8,000 international units, or IU, a day due to the risk of birth defects when taking very high amounts) and, possibly, vitamin D (400 to 800 IU is commonly recommended for bone health and other benefits).

For women, taking a prenatal vitamin six months prior to conception is recommended. When nutrients like iron, folic acid, and others are low, conception can be more difficult. We'll offer tips on how to choose a good prenatal vitamin in Chapter 8.

BOTANICAL MEDICINE

Generally, people don't need botanical medicine (also called plant or herbal medicine) on a routine basis. Unlike vitamins, minerals, and other nutrients essential to good health and to life itself, botanical substances do not occur naturally in the body. In fact, it can be argued that the body can become dependent on or habituated to certain herbs when used on a long-term basis.

Botanical medicine is very useful in treating many conditions, including several causes of infertility that you'll read about in Chapter 9. But herbal medicine is not necessary for many people trying to conceive. There are certain herbs that you should actually avoid when trying to get pregnant, which will be covered in Chapter 8.

ENVIRONMENTAL MEDICINE

Protecting the integrity of your cells and especially your DNA should be a priority when you're trying to conceive, as you'll pass along your genetic material—literally the blueprints for your child's every quality and characteristic—to the next generation. DNA is susceptible to oxidation, as mentioned earlier, and is constantly being damaged and repaired in our cells. Studies have determined that low-birth-weight babies, small or growth-restricted newborns, or preterm infants (those born before thirty-six weeks) are associated with increased oxidative DNA damage in the last three months of pregnancy.[25] Limiting the amount of environmental toxins to which you're exposed is one way to optimize your reproductive health and overall health for years to come.

Our modern world is much more toxic than the world of a hundred years ago in terms of the pollution and chemicals around us. Pesticides used to grow crops, heavy metals (like lead in old paint and mercury in contaminated fish), and chemicals common in household cleaners are among the toxins prevalent today, but best avoided. There is debate about the degree of health risk associated with some environmental contaminants, but studies have shown correlations between exposure to specific toxins and decreased fertility. Some study results have suggested that fertility levels among men are on a steady decline, and one suspected cause is toxic environmental exposure.[26]

For example, polychlorinated biphenyls, or PCBs, are potentially toxic compounds found in pesticides and elsewhere in the environment that have been shown to affect sperm quality. A study published in the journal *Human Reproduction* found that, among subjects with normal semen quality, sperm count and sperm motility were inversely related to PCB concentration. The higher the PCB concentration, the lower the sperm count and motility.[27] Another study detected PCBs in seminal plasma of infertile men but not in healthy male subjects. Sperm quantity and quality were significantly lower in the infertile men. Urban dwellers who ate fish had the highest PCB concentrations, and non–fish-eating rural dwellers had the lowest levels. The authors of the study concluded that PCBs might play a big role in the deterioration of sperm quantity and quality, with contaminated fish being the main dietary source of these toxins.[28]

Exposure to PCBs and dioxins, another class of environmental toxins, has also been shown to negatively affect fertility in women.[29] These toxins may interfere with normal growth and development in infants, too. It's still unclear exactly what the short-term and long-term effects are on babies born to parents with high levels of toxins.

Not all studies have found a link between contaminated fish and fertility, however. One study found that eating fish from the Great Lakes—which are contaminated with halogenated organics, heavy metals, and pesticides—was not associated with an increase in the amount of time it took women to get pregnant.[30] Even so, there is enough evidence of a potentially negative effect to warrant avoiding PCBs and other environmental toxins whenever possible for general health and fertility.

PCBs are considered xenoestrogens because they come from outside the body and mimic the activity of estrogens once in the body. By doing so, they modify the metabolism of natural estrogens, or compete with a form of estrogen called estradiol when binding to estrogen receptors in the body. In this way, xenoestrogens may contribute to impaired fertility, as well as early puberty and some kinds of cancer.[31]

Heavy metals contribute to infertility and should be avoided. Exposure to toxic levels of cadmium has been associated with low sperm count and volume in observation studies.[32] Lead exposure may decrease libido in men and can lead to abnormal sperm shape, reduced sperm motility, chromosomal damage, impaired prostate function, and other reproductive problems that may decrease fertility. The same study showed that, in women, lead can cause infertility, miscarriage, and other problems, including potential, varied effects on the baby.[33] Though treatment is possible, it is important to detect lead toxicity as early as possible to ensure optimal neurological functioning of the child.

Minimizing Exposure to Toxins at Work and at Home

Fortunately, there are ways to minimize your exposure to many unsavory environmental toxins. If one partner has a career in which he or she is exposed to high levels of chemicals, consider the possibility of switching from that job to one with a safer environment. Farmers, plant nursery employees, battery factory workers, and people who work around solvents and metal processing may be at risk. Working in such industries may increase the risk of exposure not only to the worker, but also to his or her family, as some pollutants can unintentionally be brought home on clothes, hair, and skin. Making the home as toxin-free as possible is especially important, considering how much time most people spend there.

Watch Your Water

The source of drinking water coming into your house should be considered. Is it public or private? Contrary to popular belief, public water supplies are often safer than those from private wells. That's because in a public system regulations exist and routine monitoring of water quality, based on the size of the system, takes place. That means water in New York City may be of higher quality than that in a rural Midwestern town. Once public water leaves the municipal treatment center and goes through the water mains, it can potentially be contaminated by bacteria and, in some cases, can pick up lead. If public water makes it to your property line safely, there usually aren't problems at the tap, unless you're in an older home with lead plumbing or lead-soldered joints.

Private wells, on the other hand, can go without testing for years; they only have to be tested when the property changes hands. Dug wells are prone to bacterial contamination and contamination from agricultural runoff (nitrates). High contaminate levels are especially common in Midwestern wells, and newborns, infants, children, and pregnant women are among the groups most vulnerable to ill effects. Drilled wells are prone to chemical contamination from petroleum products leaking from underground storage tanks, for example. Regularly testing private wells and using an effective water filter can protect you from such hazards. Find a state-approved laboratory to test your well on the Environmental Protection Agency website (see the Resources section at the back of this book).

Bottled water is often fine to drink, but water that is packaged and sold within the same state (more than half of the bottled water in the United States) is not regulated at all. FDA regulations do cover other kinds of bottled water, but the standards are not as stringent as those required of tap water. A nonprofit organization called NSF International certifies some bottled waters and provides information on approved varieties (see Resources for contact information).

Home water-filter units containing carbon filters are popular due to their ability to filter out organic contaminants. There is no one filter that removes all contaminants, so try to find out which contaminants are most likely to be in your water. NSF International certifies and tests home filters and the Water Quality Association offers a list of approved units for removing a variety of contaminants. (See Resources for contact information and other useful websites.)

Another thing you can do to keep your drinking water safer is to avoid dumping toxic household chemicals and automotive products down the drain, so that you don't end up drinking them later. To order the Environmental Protection Agency's pamphlet on home water filters, call the Environmental Resource Information Center at 1-800-276-0462 and ask for document #R-091.

Get Rid of Gases

Indoors, problems can arise from combustion gases, including environmental tobacco smoke (horrible for everyone in the house and linked to increased pneumonia, bronchitis, and other respiratory problems in children) and carbon monoxide from heating and cooking devices that aren't well ventilated. Even moderately high levels of carbon monoxide may be an underlying cause of cerebrovascular disease, though that association usually goes unnoticed. Carbon monoxide can also cause flulike feelings and usually comes from a defective heating system or an unventilated gas stove.

Another potentially dangerous gas from heating systems is nitrogen dioxide, which irritates the respiratory tract and can be a problem if the draft doesn't draw well or there are cracks in the chimney. Nitrogen dioxide may even contribute to emphysema. The Environmental Protection Agency (EPA) recommends using exhaust fans over gas stoves and ranges, keeping the burners properly adjusted, using woodstoves that meet EPA emission standards, and having furnaces, flues, and chimneys regularly inspected and maintained to reduce exposure to combustion gases at home. Robert K. McLellan, M.D., M.P.H., an environmental physician and Medical Director of Equinox Health and Healing in Portsmouth, New Hampshire, recommends asking the gas company to turn off gas pilot lights, advocates cleaning and maintaining your chimney annually, and warns against idling cars in garages.

According to the federal government, people should measure radon levels in their homes. That's because this colorless, odorless, radioactive gas—the most common source of which is uranium in soil or rock underneath the home—can cause lung cancer. Radon gas is released when uranium breaks down naturally and enters through dirt floors, floor drains, and cracks in concrete walls. Radon air concentration indoors then tends to build up, making exposure potentially dangerous through inhalation. According to the EPA, radon causes an estimated 14,000 deaths each year in the United States.

Using do-it-yourself, inexpensive test kits can help you find out if radon is a problem. Choose a state-certified kit or one that meets the standards of a national

radon proficiency program. There are also trained contractors who do radon testing. (See Resources for more information on the EPA's excellent indoor air-quality
guide.) Skilled contractors can help treat radon problems, too. Well water is sometimes a source of radon and can be remedied. Call the EPA Drinking Water Hotline
at 1-800-426-4791 to learn more.

Seek Out Safer Household Cleaners

The potent stuff you use to scrub the floor and clean the kitchen counter can pose
serious health risks. Some can cause irritation on the skin of sensitive people, and
everyone should know by now that such products can be very dangerous if ingested
or if the eyes or other sensitive areas are exposed. But there are safety concerns
beyond the obvious. Ingredients found in all-purpose cleaners (diethanolamine, or
DEA; morpholine; and triethanolamine, or TEA) may react with nitrites used as
preservatives to form nitrosamines that are carcinogenic, or cancer-causing, according to the authors of *The Safe Shopper's Bible*.[34] These nitrosamines can penetrate
the skin. Products containing butyl cellosolve, unspecified artificial colors, and all
aerosols are also best avoided.

Safe alternatives to questionable cleaning products abound in health food
stores, and you can even use vinegar, baking soda, and other simple and safe ingredients to make your own effective cleaners (see "Homework: Natural Alternatives
for Household Cleaning" on page 44). Use essential oils to freshen the air rather
than dangerous artificial fragrances; many also have antibacterial effects. Several
books rate brands of household products on safety and effectiveness. Check your
library or health food store for them.

If you do use products that might cause irritation, wear plastic gloves and crack
a window. Do not mix chlorine cleaners or bleach with other cleaning products,
ammonia, or acids. Keep products away from kids and find out if there is a community center in your area for collection of toxic household waste so you can safely
dispose of what you no longer want or need.

Avoid VOCs

Volatile organic compounds, or VOCs, can be expelled from the materials containing them. This means that synthetic carpeting, kitchen cabinets, wall paneling,
paints, adhesives, and other common household materials release VOCs into the air,
which can lead to sinus and lung irritation. Dry-cleaning fluids that remain on
clothes are another culprit. If they emit a strong smell, demand that the dry cleaner
remedy the situation. Formaldehyde from modern building materials and other
household products (permanent-press fabrics, particle board, carpet, paints, sham-

poos, plastics, insulation, and tobacco smoke, for example) is one of the most well-researched VOCs, but, according to John Bower in his book *The Healthy House, IV,* there are hundreds of others we currently know little about.[35]

Formaldehyde alone can cause burning eyes, headaches, asthma attacks, nausea, and breathing difficulty. It has also caused cancer in animals and may do the same in humans. Most formaldehyde is released within the first year of the product's life, so exposure at least decreases over time.

Sometimes even if the VOC source is removed from the house, VOCs have been absorbed by and may be released from another material that remains—curtains, wood, furniture, gypsum wallboard, and carpet, for example. Choosing building materials that don't contain VOC is best. If you already have them, carefully removing the source of VOCs is ideal, but not always practical and can be cost-prohibitive. See *The Healthy House* and the EPA website for more information about dealing with VOCs. Several companies now specialize in safer building materials, and Bower's book and others can steer you in the right direction.

Be Aware of Other Toxins Lurking at Home

From the early 1900s through the late 1970s, asbestos was used in insulation, drywall joint compound, and floor tile made of vinyl. Now we know that this mineral is dangerous when its particles are inhaled; it causes a lung disease called asbestosis, as well as cancer. When a product containing asbestos begins to disintegrate or is disturbed, particles become airborne and can be inhaled. When it is solid and not breaking down, it's unlikely to make you sick. Sometimes it's safer to seal off asbestos with an encapsulating sealant than to remove it. Before the dangers of asbestos were realized, asbestos workers not only were exposed to these dangerous pollutants but brought the danger home to their loved ones on their clothes and body. Unfortunately, it was decades later before the link between health problems and asbestos was appreciated by the public. The EPA has a booklet about asbestos and its removal, or you can call the Consumer Product Safety Commission (1-800-638-CPSC) or your state health department for more information.

Heavy metals pose serious health risks, too. Lead paint is still found in homes, and when it erodes from windows as they are opened and shut over the years, tiny chips can find their way onto children's hands and into their mouths, leading to lead poisoning. Have your house tested for lead paint if you have children younger than six years old. If you live in a house with lead paint, have any children aged eighteen months to five years old tested. All lead-covered surfaces that kids can reach should be specially treated by a professional to remove the lead or cover it with a permanent barrier, not merely coated with more paint.

Mercury and cadmium are other dangerous metals found in some paints, and mercury from broken thermometers can be dangerous when it evaporates and contaminates the air, possibly resulting in nervous system damage and other organ damage. Arsenic is also dangerous to health, and it may be found in treated lumber used for decks and railings that is sometimes described as "salt-treated," referring to arsenic salt. Seek out wood for building projects that is free from metals and other potential contaminants.

To decrease the amount of airborne particulates containing dust, other allergens, and potential contaminants in your home, always vacuum instead of dry sweeping, recommends Margee Virant, Vice President of Operational Development of The Maids International, a maid service franchiser that specializes in cleaning for health. Sweeping just sends particles back into the air, while vacuuming (use a vacuum with HEPA filters) takes particles out of the environment and traps them. Use microfiber cloths instead of feather dusters for the same reason.

Change your furnace filters regularly and get rid of clutter. Open a door or window often to get fresh air in and dirty air out, even if it's just a crack during cold weather. Many air filters are available, but limiting contaminants and allergens in the air in the first place is preferred, as is adequate ventilation. See the EPA's guide to indoor air quality for information on the complex topic of choosing air filters. Exposure to dust mites, which many people are allergic to, can be reduced in bedding by using tightly woven cotton mattress and pillow casings. Head to the health food store for natural and safer alternatives to DEET-containing insect repellents and other personal care products that might cause problems.

Helpful tips to avoid toxins in food include buying organic food to avoid pesticide exposure; storing food properly; cleaning all utensils, cutting boards, and preparation areas thoroughly with very hot water; washing produce carefully; avoiding fish associated with high metal contamination; and cooking food (especially meat and eggs) at temperatures high enough to kill any potential pathogens.

Finally, don't allow smoking indoors. As a clinician, I can testify that I have lost patients to secondhand smoke. These people hadn't smoked a day in their lives, yet their spouses did and they died of lung cancer. Children can get asthma, ear infections, respiratory illnesses, and heavy-metal poisoning from cadmium and other toxic substances found in cigarette smoke. If you smoke, always smoke outside. But the best thing you can do is to stop smoking altogether because even if you smoke outdoors, your clothes harbor pollutants, and your baby can be passively exposed to them when you handle him or her. Also, your clothes leave a residue of pollutants in the washing machine that will cling to other clothes.

Homework

NATURAL ALTERNATIVES FOR HOUSEHOLD CLEANING

Ready to go natural when it comes to cleaning? Here are some eco-friendly and economical alternatives to conventional and potentially harmful cleaning products. (Hang a copy of this list in a kitchen cupboard for easy reference.)

✿ Cut grease and stubborn leftover food from dishes and glasses by putting a few lemon slices or a tablespoon of vinegar into a sink of soapy water.

✿ Remove scuff marks from vinyl floors by scouring with baking soda.

✿ Add a small square of aluminum foil and boiling water to baking soda to wash silver.

✿ Remove toilet-bowl rings with a paste made of baking soda and vinegar.

✿ Polish chrome using a small amount of baby oil on a soft, clean cloth.

✿ Remove hard-water spots from glasses and crystal by soaking them in a sink filled with near-boiling water and 2 cups of white vinegar for five to ten minutes. (Don't let crystal touch crystal; it will scratch.)

✿ Remove cleaning-product buildup from windows by rubbing them with a cotton swab of rubbing alcohol, then wash with a mix of 2 tablespoons vinegar and 1 quart of water.

✿ Get spots out of clothing, carpet, and upholstery with a healthy dose of club soda or lemon juice.

✿ Polish wood with three parts olive oil and one part white vinegar.

✿ Clear a clogged drain with a half cup of baking soda and a half cup of vinegar. Let that sit for five minutes, then flush with boiling water.

✿ Use a 50/50 vinegar and water mix to take soot off of fireplace doors; wipe them clean with old newspaper.

✿ Use toothpaste to clean porcelain, chrome, and stone surfaces.

Additional Strategies to Limit Your Exposure to Toxins

Here are a few more ways you can reduce your risk of exposure to dangerous environmental toxins as you strive for optimal health:

- If working or driving in polluted cities, keep your windows closed during the commute. Also keep windows closed at work and home during air-quality alerts and rush hour.

- If there is a fireplace or field in your vicinity where burning is being done, minimize exposure. Many people end up burning things that release very dangerous byproducts when heated.

- Don't exercise on busy streets polluted by cars, trucks, and other vehicles.

- Don't pick fruit, berries, or other edibles by busy streets, potentially polluted creeks, or anywhere you suspect the plants may have been sprayed or contaminated. When in doubt, keep your hands in your pockets and your lips tightly sealed.

- Remember that you can absorb many things through your skin. Wear protective gloves when working with chemicals.

- The body can get heavily burdened when you breathe in toxic substances. Work on crafts or other projects involving exposure to smells and vapors only in a very well-ventilated area, or wear an appropriate, approved respiratory device.

Meet the Challenge with Courage, Not Fear

All this information isn't meant to scare you into living life in a bubble. As we've made clear, you can do many things to make your body and your home healthier. Like getting the best nutrition and taking care of your relationship and mental health, decreasing your exposure to environmental toxins will improve your health and potentially boost your fertility.

As a preventive measure, flip through the yellow pages to find a home inspector to test for radon, lead, drinking water contaminants, or whatever else concerns you. Seek out an occupational and environmental medicine physician if you think you may be ill from something inside your home or workplace. The American College of Occupational and Environmental Medicine (see Resources) can help you find an experienced practitioner. With a little effort and education, your home can be a safe haven for you and your family.

MORE TIPS FOR A HEALTHY LIFESTYLE

Here are some more simple strategies for both men and women that may help optimize fertility.

- **Keep cool, fellas.** Maintaining an ideal scrotal temperature (94–96 degrees Fahrenheit) is necessary for normal sperm production. At higher temperatures, sperm production becomes limited or stops entirely. Men should avoid hot tubs and saunas, opt for boxers over briefs, and avoid wearing tight pants. Whether or not wearing boxers rather than briefs truly affects fertility is open for debate, but it certainly can't hurt. Exercises associated with increased scrotal temperature include rowing machines, simulated cross-country ski machines, jogging, and treadmills. Let the testicles hang freely to cool down after exercising. Taking a cold shower is another strategy that infertile men may want to try. A testicular hypothermia device, somewhat like a jock strap that circulates cold water, can be concealed under clothes during the day.

- **Exercise moderately and regularly, but not too intensely.** A healthy exercise routine for men and women has many benefits, but exercising intensely for an extended time may hinder fertility for various reasons. Brisk walking and yoga are options, though hot yoga or anything that causes stress or increased chance of detoxification should be avoided. Examples are excess sweating and heat, including exercising outdoors on hot days, saunas, and so on. Opt for exercise that allows you to carry on a casual conversation simultaneously without gasping for air. That way, you are more likely to stay in your aerobic exercise mode and not cause unnecessary buildup of anaerobic metabolites like lactic acid. Aim for a session of moderate exercise lasting twenty to thirty minutes, but not more than forty to forty-five minutes, two to three times a week. A daily walking routine of twenty minutes at a mild and relaxing pace is fine, as well.

  Pregnant women should avoid doing anything that might either dehydrate the body or release toxins stored in fat tissues that will then enter the circulation system and possibly expose the baby. Another recommendation is steering clear of any exercise that causes you to increase intra-abdominal pressure, such as lifting weights or exercises that cause an intense bearing down or cause you to hold your breath.

- **Work with your doctor to adjust prescription drug intake, if possible.** Nonsteroidal anti-inflammatory drugs (NSAIDs) have been linked to infertility in women, and these and other drugs may hinder fertility in men, too. Steroids taken by athletes to bulk up and Azulfidine for irritable bowel disease can interfere with normal sperm production. Talk with your prescribing doctor to determine if it's possible to decrease or discontinue any drugs you are taking that may decrease fertility. Once you stop taking the medication (with your doctor's approval), it takes three to six months for sperm production to return to normal levels. It is imperative that you work with a practitioner to carefully adjust your medication.

- **If you smoke or use illegal drugs, quit.** Cigarette smoke, as well as marijuana and cocaine usage, damages tiny blood vessels that supply blood to the penis, decreasing sexual functioning. Cigarette smoking also depletes vitamins and minerals, compromising health in men, women, and fetuses. In addition, researchers have determined that chemicals in tobacco increase the risk of low birth weight, miscarriage, and birth defects.

- **Avoid using vaginal lubricants, if possible.** Commercial vaginal lubricants significantly impair sperm motility, which is important for fertilization. In a study testing popular lubricants (K-Y Jelly, Astroglide, Replens, and Touch) and vegetable oil products used as lubricants, the commercial lubricants inhibited sperm motility by 60 to 100 percent after sixty minutes of incubation. Canola oil had no detrimental effect on sperm motility.[36] (Check with your physician prior to using lubricant containing canola oil.) Unscented vitamin E and mineral oils are other acceptable alternatives.

MAKE CHANGES NOW FOR A FERTILE FUTURE

Trying to take in all the information in this chapter may feel overwhelming; we've covered a lot. But it's vitally important to your health and to that of a potential baby that you invest the time and energy to optimize your health by tending to your relationship with your spouse, making your environment as safe as possible, eating well, taking a good multivitamin, and adopting healthy lifestyle habits. Ideally, you should implement these changes at least a few months before you try to conceive, since it takes time to reap the rewards of good habits. For example, it takes sperm three to six months to change significantly as a result of diet and lifestyle adjustments. As you'll see from the success stories we've included throughout the following chapters, the effort often does pay off.

SUMMARY OF FERTILITY-FRIENDLY TIPS FOR MEN AND WOMEN

- Take stock of your relationship health, and talk with your partner and friends who have children about expectations and lifestyle changes that go with having a baby.

- Keep your weight within a healthy range and talk to your doctor about gaining or losing weight, if necessary.

- Eat a healthy diet heavy on plant foods (organic whenever possible).

- Limit saturated fat and other bad fats; focus on good fats from vegetable and fish sources.

- Choose a good daily multivitamin and mineral supplement.

- Limit exposure to harmful toxins in the environment by using natural cleaning products and having your home tested for toxins in the water and air.

- Exercise moderately and regularly, but not too intensely. Yoga is one form of exercise that can help reduce stress (though hot yoga should be avoided when trying to get pregnant).

3

Whole-Person Health Care: A Starting Point for You and Your Physician

By now you realize the importance of being as healthy as possible when trying to conceive—for your own well-being, in order to maximize your odds of conception, and to increase the likelihood of giving birth to a healthy baby. In earlier chapters, we helped lay the groundwork for a healthy foundation with diet and lifestyle tips. Another important way to ensure that you are in the best possible health is to undergo a series of medical tests with your healthcare practitioner. In this chapter we'll cover initial tests and physical exams that all couples should have prior to conception and tests recommended for couples who haven't yet gotten pregnant after actively trying. We'll also give some pointers to assist you in finding the right doctor, whether it's a reproductive endocrinologist, a naturopathic physician, or both.

INITIAL TESTS FOR ALL COUPLES

First and foremost, make sure you are in good general health before trying to get pregnant. The following tests are recommended for all health-conscious people on an annual basis, regardless of whether or not they want to become pregnant. A willingness to conceive makes these tests even more important. Both naturopathic doctors (N.D.s) and conventional medical doctors (M.D.s) can order these tests.

Chemistry Panel

Just like its name, this test measures your body's very basic biochemical health. One simple tube of blood is all that's needed. The test should include the following:

1. **Glucose (blood sugar):** Low glucose levels suggest hypoglycemia, while high numbers can suggest diabetes.

2. **BUN (blood urea nitrogen):** A high BUN level suggests illness, possible liver problems, excess adrenal function, and other potential problems.

3. **Creatinine:** Levels of this waste product reflect how well the kidneys are working.

4. **Sodium (Na):** High sodium levels can indicate too much salt intake and a link to high blood pressure in some people. Lower-than-normal levels can contribute to fatigue and muscle weakness.

5. **Potassium (K):** High potassium levels (a condition called hyperkalemia) can result in muscle weakness, diarrhea, and heart problems related to changes in electrical impulse. Lower-than-normal levels of potassium (hypokalemia) can lead to muscle weakness, heart arrhythmias, breathing problems, nausea, and other conditions.

6. **Chloride (Cl):** This is the negatively charged partner of sodium (Na). Chloride and sodium are usually consumed together in the form of table salt (NaCl). Like sodium, potassium, and other electrolytes, chloride helps maintain the proper balance and concentration of body fluids and helps to regulate acid-to-base balance. Body fluids must constantly contain a balance of acids and bases. (Acids are substances that dissociate into one or more hydrogen ions and one or more anions, or negative ions; they are proton donors. Bases dissociate into one or more hydroxide ions or one or more cations, or positive ions; they are proton acceptors.)

7. **Uric acid:** High levels of uric acid can lead to a form of arthritis called gout and can result from eating too much shellfish, organ meat, or alcohol, along with other causes.

8. **Cholesterol:** High levels of cholesterol can signify increased risk of heart disease, but levels that are too low can mean that steroidal hormones such as estrogen, testosterone, progesterone, and others made from cholesterol may also be lower than ideal. A total cholesterol level of 140 to 199 milligrams per deciliter (mg/dl) is considered healthy in conventional medicine. A total of 140 to 175 mg/dl is ideal in naturopathic terms. The ratio of HDL to LDL cholesterol is also important (more on this below).

9. **HDL:** A high ratio of high-density lipoproteins (HDL), often referred to as "good" cholesterol, to low-density lipoproteins (LDL), often called "bad" cholesterol, is desirable. (To distinguish between HDL and LDL, think of the "H" as a highway patrol, guarding the highways, that is blood vessels, of your body from damage.) Regular exercise, low stress levels, and a diet high in fiber and low in hydrogenated oils from processed foods help boost HDL levels. For

men, HDL levels between 37 and 70 mg/dl are considered healthy. In naturopathic terms, levels from 50 to 75 mg/dl and up are ideal. For women, the healthy conventional range is 40 to 85 mg/dl and the naturopathic range is 50 to 100 mg/dl.

10. **LDL:** The "bad" cholesterol contributes to clogging arteries. Low-density lipoprotein (LDL) is susceptible to lipid peroxidation (free-radical damage to fats), which sets the stage for a series of events that lead to arterial blockage and, ultimately, a heart attack. (Think of "L" for litterbug, as LDL jams up the blood flow in your blood vessels.) The conventional healthy level of LDL is less than 130 mg/dl and the healthy naturopathic level is less than 90 mg/dl. Doctors also consider the ratio of LDL to HDL cholesterol levels in determining heart disease risk. The higher the ratio of HDL to LDL, the better.

11. **Total protein:** This number provides clues about how much protein you are eating, absorbing, using, and whether or not you are getting enough. Too much protein may be hard on the kidneys, because excess protein requires the kidneys to work harder. Too little protein may hinder fertility and prevent the body from repairing itself adequately. For example, protein helps muscles recover from working out and aids in wound healing from injury and everyday wear and tear. Protein also provides the building blocks for a baby's development.

12. **Albumin:** This protein is made in the liver. You need sufficient total protein as a raw ingredient for the creation of albumin. Albumin is critical to prevent the fluid in your body from seeping out of the blood vessels, which is one cause of edema (swelling due to fluid collecting in the tissues), such as in the feet and ankles.

13. **Globulin:** Globulin is another important protein with multiple functions, including immunoglobulin function (which means it plays a role in immunity).

14. **AST, ALT, GGT, and bilirubin:** AST, ALT, and GGT are enzymes most commonly associated with the liver, and high bilirubin levels suggest liver problems. Levels of these enzymes and bilirubin help measure the general health level of your liver, and they can be elevated in such conditions as hemolytic anemia, in which blood cells rupture. These levels can be elevated for other reasons, such as due to the liver disease hepatitis.

15. **Alkaline phosphatase:** Alkaline phosphatase is often referred to as a bone enzyme, and it is normally higher in growing children than in adults because active bone growth causes higher levels. High levels of bone enzyme in adults,

however, can be a sign of bone disease (such as bone cancer) and fractures, but it can also be elevated for other reasons.

16. **TSH:** Thyroid-stimulating hormone (TSH) is used to measure thyroid levels. In an ideal blood panel, however, thyroxine, T3 uptake, and free thyroxine levels are also measured. Think of thyroid levels of thyroxine and TSH as having a boss-to-employee relationship: Thyroxine (thyroid hormone) is like an employee in a factory; it's what actually gets the job done. TSH is like the supervisor, making sure there's no loafing on the job. If thyroid hormone levels are low, the TSH (boss) starts raising its voice to be heard, and the level of TSH in the body becomes elevated. If there's overproduction, then TSH falls asleep because it's not needed; this occurs in Graves' disease (hyperthyroidism), from which Barbara Bush suffered. The TSH level also gauges how well the pituitary gland—which monitors TSH secretion—is working. Yet counting totally on the TSH assumes that the pituitary is on the job and able to accommodate changes in circulating thyroid, which it may not be able to do if there is a disease of the pituitary gland. High thyroid levels are often associated with increased blood pressure, elevated body temperature, increased pulse, weight loss, and other signs of a hyperactive body, such as sleeplessness and fast bowel activity. The opposite is true for low thyroid levels, which can cause slower thinking, dry skin, constipation, low body temperature, low blood pressure, and low pulse.

CBC Testing

Complete blood count, or CBC, is considered a must because it gives clear insight into immune function within your body and the health of your red blood cell profile.

White blood cell count, or WBC, is a measure of the total number of various white blood cells within the body's army. Neutrophils, lymphocytes, macrophages, phagocytes, eosinophils, basophils, and monocytes are all white blood cells and each has a special function. (Macrophages and phagocytes, however, aren't measured in WBC testing.) Their roles range from hand-to-hand combat against invading bacteria and viruses to the body's equivalent of biological warfare. The body works like the scanner in the grocery store: the immune system looks at the protein codes on the cells that go by, and if it determines that a bacteria, virus, or other substance has entered the body, it calls out the troops. Neutrophils are the forces that predominantly combat a bacterial invasion, and lymphocytes take care of viral problems. So high levels of neutrophils suggest a bacterial infection; high levels of lymphocytes indicate a viral infection. Immune cells called macrophages and phagocytes act like Pac-Man, engulfing and gobbling up the enemy—anything the body recognizes as nonself, or foreign.

Red blood cell count, or RBC, gives insight into the body's ability to effectively and efficiently deliver oxygen and nutrients throughout the body. It also helps determine whether or not you have enough iron in your body. If you are anemic, it could mean that you are deficient in iron or another nutrient, such as folic acid, which should be remedied before getting pregnant. Iron deficiency might be responsible for miscarriage, preterm labor, fetal malformations, and intrauterine growth retardation.[1] Folic acid deficiency can cause neural tube defects like spina bifida in offspring, which is why women of childbearing age are encouraged to take a folic acid supplement and why many foods are now fortified with this B vitamin.

STD Testing

It's a good idea to undergo testing to make sure you haven't been exposed to a sexually transmitted disease (STD). The vast majority of these tests are done with blood work and by asking patients about symptoms; occasionally, a swab is used to collect a specimen of tissue from the reproductive tract. Not all STDs present symptoms, so you could have such a disease but have no symptoms, which makes testing all the more vital. Venereal diseases including gonorrhea, syphilis, and genital herpes are all STDs, and AIDS (acquired immunodeficiency syndrome) is a particularly serious STD.

STDs can inhibit fertility by causing obstruction of either male or female reproductive ducts; they can also cause pregnancy wastage, including miscarriages and stillbirths, and neonatal deaths (during the first four weeks after birth).[2] In women, organisms moving up from the vagina and cervix can infect the Fallopian tubes, uterus, ovaries, and surrounding structures. Scars from infections form in and around the tubes, potentially preventing sperm from reaching the egg in the tube or preventing the tube from moving the fertilized egg to the uterus. This situation can result in a troublesome tubal pregnancy.

Nutritional Physical and Questionnaire

Your body creates clues about what is going on within the trillions of cells that make it up. Just as we look at a person's pet and say they have a healthy coat, our hair, nails, teeth, and skin reflect our health. For example, dry skin might suggest low thyroid disease, lack of sufficient nutrients like essential fatty acids, or possibly inadequate water intake. Dark circles under the eyes, often referred to as allergic shiners, suggest food allergies or may point to poor digestion, constipation, or other conditions. A diagonal crease in your earlobe might be the sign of heart disease. Some practitioners believe there is a strong correlation between deterioration of the capillaries (blood vessels) in the ears and what is going on in the rest of the body.

The section below lists some considerations that you may want to discuss with your physician during your routine physical exam. A visit to a nutritionally oriented physician will often include a standard physical exam and at the same time the physician will be looking for signs of potential nutritional or health conditions that would not typically be picked up by the untrained eye. For example, an average healthcare provider might look into a patient's eyes as part of a normal physical and dismiss the dark circles under them as normal since so many people suffer from poor digestion and allergies. A nutritionally oriented physician, on the other hand, would consider dark circles a clue to specific health problems to be solved.

NUTRITIONAL CONSIDERATIONS DURING A PHYSICAL EXAM

Modified and reprinted with permission from *Medical Nutrition from Marz,* 2nd Edition, Omni-Press, Portland, Oregon, 1997; 500–501.

Note to Readers: The following information is intended as educational and is not designed to be either diagnostic or a suggestion of treatment. Only you and your physician working together as a team can determine what is best for you. Please share these thoughts with your physician.

If you are pregnant or wish to become pregnant, working with your physician is even more important to ensure that the dosages and choice of supplements that you wish to take are also good for your desired little one.

1. Blood Pressure

- Ideally 120/80 mm Hg or slightly below.
- With increased blood pressure, consider essential fatty acids (EFAs), magnesium, calcium, and potassium.
- With decreased blood pressure, consider anemia, hypothyroid, hypoadrenal (subclinical).

2. Head

Dry hair: Consider hypothyroidism and low essential fatty acids and zinc.
Premature graying: Consider calcium deficiency.

Hair loss: Consider poor circulation, parasitic infection, malnutrition, heavy metal toxicity, etc. Possible supplements: folic acid, B_6, B_{12} (B complex), and zinc.

Dandruff: Excess intake of carbohydrates and insufficient essential fatty acids and minerals. Possible supplements: EFAs, antioxidants (especially selenium), and vitamin B_6 and/or B complex.

3. Face

Seborrheic dermatitis: Shiny and scaly forehead with yellow greasy look that can extend into eyebrows, down nose, cheeks, chest. Possible treatment consideration: vitamin B_6 or B complex, EFAs.

Vertical creases: Vertical creases of forehead near midline may be correlated with duodenal ulcers, especially when accompanied with upper abdomen discomfort.

Acne: Face and back:

Limit sugar, increase green leafy vegetables daily.

Consider zinc, essential fatty acids, avoiding food allergies, and presence of sufficient stomach acidity.

Dilated capillaries: Cheeks and nose:

Consider too much alcohol has been consumed or too little stomach acidity.

Acne rosacea: Redness of cheeks and forehead along with pimples. Consider food allergies, insufficient stomach acidity, sensitivity to carbohydrates. Possible presence of *H. pylori,* a bacteria in the stomach linked to stomach ulcers.

4. Ears

Diagonal ear lobe creases: Strong correlation with cardiovascular disease.

Ear wax: When excess and dark may be sign of essential fatty acid deficiency.

Ear drum: When fluid appears to be present behind eardrum, may be due to allergies such as dairy or wheat allergy.

Ménière's disease: Can be strongly correlated with food and environmental allergies, among other causes.

Ringing: May be due to food allergies, cardiovascular disease, aspirin toxicity.

5. Neck

Skin tag: Multiple pigmented skin tags often correlate with abnormal blood sugars (also under arms).

Lymph nodes: Swollen lymph nodes should be examined by a physician and are not considered normal. There are many causes, including allergies, infection, and more serious illnesses.

6. Skin

Dry: Hypothyroidism, essential fatty acids, or too much soap or chlorinated water.

Follicular hyperkeratosis: Small bumps at base hair follicles on back of arms and anterior thighs. EFAs may help.

Slow wound healing: May be due to diabetes, deficiency of vitamin C, zinc, protein, and essential fatty acids.

Yeast/Fungus: Consider imbalanced blood sugar, also rule out *Candida albicans.*

Bruising easily: Consider supplementation with vitamin C with bioflavonoids, vitamin K (especially with poor digestive absorption or following antibiotics).

7. Nails

Flat angle and spooning: Iron deficiency is a common cause.

Soft poor growth: Often due to one or more mineral deficiencies.

Hard nails or cuticle inflammation: May be due to zinc deficiency.

Brittle nails: Hypothyroid, decreased stomach acidity, mineral deficiency, or protein deficiency.

Ridging: Consider lack of mineral absorption or consumption. Can also be correlated with eczema and/or psoriasis.

8. Hands

Eczema: Consider allergies and supplementation of zinc, B_6, and EFAs.

Hang nails: Consider zinc supplementation.

Cracking tips of fingers: Consider zinc supplementation.

Cold hands: Hypothyroid, cardiovascular disease, allergies. Consider Raynaud's disease and anemia. Treatments can include ginkgo, niacin, vitamin E, and treating the underlying health condition.

Dupuytren's contracture: Tissue thickening on palm along tendon of fourth finger. Treatment with vitamin E. Consider blood sugar imbalance.

Ulnar deviation: Shifting of fingers that can result from rheumatoid arthritis.

9. Eyes

Dark circles under eyes: Allergic shiners. Avoid food allergens. Consider blepharitis, conjunctivitis, xanthomas, retinol hemmorhages.

Floaters: Anemia, deficiency of vitamin C, vitamin K, bioflavonoids.

10. Nose

Salute sign: Horizontal lines across bridge of nose. Consider allergies and inflamed sinuses, routine rubbing of nose.

Intranasal polyps: Allergies or salicylate sensitivity.

Loss of sense of smell: Can result from zinc deficiency.

Rash around nose: Consider essential fatty acids, antioxidants, and allergies. Prominent rash extending from nose to cheeks. Visit with your doctor about lupus if the rash is butterfly in shape and worsens with sun exposure or associated with joint stiffness.

11. Mouth

Teeth: Numerous mercury fillings may affect thyroid or central nervous system.

Tooth decay: Consider poor mineral absorption, such as decreased boron, silica, calcium, B_6. Avoid simple carbohydrates and practice good oral hygiene.

Periodontal disease: Deficiency of calcium, vitamin C, CoQ_{10}, bioflavonoids, zinc, and folic acid.

Bleeding gums: Consider supplementation with vitamin C, bioflavinoids, CoQ_{10}. Brush gently and avoid hard-bristle toothbrushes.

Canker sores: Allergies. Avoid gluten (found in grains), simple carbohydrates, pineapple, citrus, coffee.

Tonsils: Enlarged, commonly due to allergies (both environmental and food) and infection.

Grinding: Excess stress and allergies (also called bruxism)

Loss of sense of taste: Can be due to zinc deficiency.

Tongue: *Glossitis:* B_{12}, folate, or iron deficiency.

Geographic tongue: Allergies, B vitamin deficiencies.

Pale: Can correlate with pale eyelid linings, suggestive of iron deficiency.

Swollen tongue: With teethmarks can signify poor digestion, allergies.

12. Urogenital

Abnormal Pap: Consider supporting other treatments offered by your physicians with vitamin B_6, folic acid, and beta-carotene.

Prostate: If enlarged, consider essential fatty acids, zinc, lycopene, glycine, arginine, saw palmetto, pygeum. Always have a physical exam and PSA annually.

Breasts: If fibrocystic, consider vitamin E, essential fatty acids. Avoid caffeine and chocolate.

PHYSICAL EXAMS ALL COUPLES SHOULD UNDERGO

Both men and women should have full physical exams, including a Pap exam for women and a prostate exam for men. Pap exams determine if disease processes are going on in the cervix or possibly in the uterus. That may affect the woman's ability to conceive or carry a pregnancy. Prostate exams can point out whether a man has prostatitis (inflammation of the prostate gland), or other health conditions that need attention. It takes healthy partners to conceive a baby in an optimal environment, and the goal of achieving long-term health will keep your focus on the baby and not on curing your body if damage has taken place.

TESTS FOR COUPLES WHO SUSPECT THEY ARE INFERTILE

Basic infertility testing is designed to evaluate the following major causes, as described here by Dr. Zalman Levine, M.D., a subspecialist in reproductive endocrinology and infertility. Dr. Levine practices at the Fertility Institute of New Jersey and New York and has a special interest and expertise in infertility, advanced assisted reproductive techniques, and reproductive surgery.

- **Ovarian causes:** "Whether or not a woman ovulates can be determined by her menstrual history, basal body temperature charting, home ovulation predictor kit testing, and blood testing for progesterone levels," says Dr. Levine. "Your physician might suggest any or all of the above. Ovarian function is a bit more complicated to test, because even if a woman is ovulating, her ovarian function, or 'ovarian reserve' as this is sometimes called, might still be a problem. Ovarian reserve tends to decline in a subtle fashion with advancing age. It can be evaluated by early-cycle blood testing for various hormones like estrogen, FSH, and inhibin B, by ultrasound assessment of the size and appearance of the ovaries, or by a hormonal test called a clomiphene challenge test."

- **Fallopian tube causes:** "The initial test to evaluate whether the Fallopian tubes are open or blocked is called a hysterosalpingogram, abbreviated HSG," says Dr. Levine. "This test is an x-ray of the Fallopian tubes, which is done by inserting a speculum into the vagina and injecting a special dye into the cervix. This dye fills up the uterus and spills out into the Fallopian tubes. If the tubes are open, the dye, which is harmless and shows up clearly on x-rays, will fill up the tubes and spill out from the ends into the woman's abdomen. Because the dye fills the uterus before entering the Fallopian tubes, the contours of the uterus can also be seen on the x-ray, which is also informative. A woman undergoing this test should expect to feel cramping because the dye irritates the uterus. Because the cramping can be very severe and painful for some women,

I recommend that anyone undergoing this test should consult her physician about taking a maximal dose of an anti-cramping agent like ibuprofen an hour before the test."

- **Male causes:** "To evaluate the sperm, the test of choice is a semen analysis in which an ejaculate of semen is examined microscopically in the lab," says Dr. Levine. "Some important parameters the lab looks for are how many sperm there are, how motile they are, and how normal they look. Ideally, the ejaculate should be produced for analysis after no fewer than three days but no more than seven days of abstinence to maximize the parameters, and ideally the analysis should take place soon after the ejaculation occurs. The analysis should be done by a lab experienced in sperm testing. If the semen analysis is abnormal, it will be repeated. If persistently abnormal, further testing and evaluation of the man may be warranted."

FINDING THE RIGHT DOCTOR

Your obstetrician-gynecologist (ob-gyn), internist, or family doctor can probably initiate help if you've been trying to get pregnant for at least six months and you're thirty-five or older, or if you're younger and have been trying for a year without success (this is especially true for women). Ob-gyns can conduct basic tests, including monitoring hormone levels, pelvic exams, and charting basal body temperature, among others. For men, urologists can order tests to determine sperm quality, do a semen analysis, measure hormone levels, and look for varicose veins in the scrotum (varicoceles). Andrologists specialize in male reproductive function with a focus on aspects like semen or hormones, as opposed to anatomical problems. If early treatment measures aren't successful after a few months or if an evaluation uncovers a problem beyond that doctor's expertise, he or she can likely refer you to a reproductive endocrinologist.

A reproductive endocrinologist is a specialist in the evaluation and treatment of infertility. These specialists spend eleven years, including medical school, studying the science and art of reproductive medicine. "They have the highest level of expertise in both the medical and the surgical aspects of the field," notes Dr. Levine. He advises couples to choose a physician with whom they feel comfortable and who provides an office environment that is highly supportive, personalized, and professional. Most specialists like both partners to come in for the first appointment. "As a reproductive endocrinologist," says Dr. Levine, "I feel strongly that treatment goals for the individual couple must be established." Couples and their doctors should work together to make sure everyone has a clear sense of the goals.

Questions you and your doctor should consider, suggests Dr. Levine, include the following: What are you trying to accomplish with certain medications? If you don't ovulate, is the goal to help you ovulate a single egg like anyone else? Or if you have unexplained infertility, do you need superovulation (the release of two or more eggs) to achieve pregnancy?

Above all, the established goals must be pursued during treatment. "It's easy for individual goals for couples to get lost in the rush of monitoring, but it's critical for physicians and patients to maintain personalized care and not to lose sight of personalized treatment goals [from] day to day," stresses Dr. Levine.

If you choose to work with a naturopathic doctor, either alone or in tandem with a reproductive endocrinologist, the American Association of Naturopathic Physicians website (www.naturopathic.org) is an excellent resource. There you can learn more about naturopathic medicine and even locate a licensed, qualified doctor in your area.

Licensed naturopathic physicians (N.D.s) are educated in the same basic sciences as M.D.s at one of the four-year, graduate-level naturopathic medical schools. In addition, they study nontoxic and holistic therapies with a focus on preventing disease and optimizing wellness. Naturopathic physicians must complete four years of training in various types of medicine—basic Chinese, homeopathic, botanical, and physical—as well as clinical nutrition, psychology, counseling, and conventional drug prescribing. Then they must pass rigorous professional board exams to be licensed by a jurisdiction or state as a primary-care general-practice physician, and their specific scope of practice is defined by state law. Thirteen states, along with the United States territories of Puerto Rico and the Virgin Islands, have licensing laws for N.D.s. In addition to meeting educational requirements and passing

States That License Naturopathic Physicians

As of April 2004, the following states, as well as the United States territories of Puerto Rico and the Virgin Islands, have licensing laws for naturopathic physicians:

✿ Alaska	✿ Kansas	✿ Oregon
✿ Arizona	✿ Maine	✿ Utah
✿ California	✿ Montana	✿ Vermont
✿ Connecticut	✿ New Hampshire	✿ Washington
✿ Hawaii		

board exams, licensed N.D.s must fulfill continuing education requirements mandated by the state each year.

When you're looking for a naturopathic physician, it's best, if you can't get a referral from a friend, to ask prospects where they graduated from. Bastyr University, Bridgeport University, the National College of Naturopathic Medicine, the Southwest College of Naturopathic Medicine, and the Canadian College of Naturopathic Medicine are well-established, respected naturopathic schools. Practitioners may have varying degrees of expertise, but an N.D. who has graduated from one of those schools will be very broadly and reliably trained. Just because a practitioner says he or she graduated from another accredited college doesn't mean that school has a four-year program that trains primary-care physicians.

Naturopathic medicine differs from conventional medicine in that it focuses on whole-patient wellness. Naturopathic physicians seek the underlying cause of a patient's condition, as opposed to just treating the symptoms. The question an N.D. asks is "Why did this patient get sick in the first place?" "Susceptibility," a term often used by N.D.'s, refers to why a person succumbed to an illness or condition. That kind of questioning can offer insights into a given health problem, as well as enlightenment about global health concerns. It also guides the practitioner to the root cause of the illness. Just as lopping off the top of a dandelion doesn't produce a healthy lawn—the dandelion will spring up again—treating just the symptoms of an illness and not dealing with the root cause rarely solves the problem.

Naturopathic medicine is custom-tailored to the patient and emphasizes prevention of health problems. N.D.s work with doctors in other branches of medicine and also refer patients to various specialists for treatment when it's appropriate. For example, if a person has low thyroid hormone levels, an N.D. could choose to send a complex case to an endocrinologist (a specialist in hormones) to draw on that doctor's expertise, just as a family doctor would. Naturopathic strategies alone are certainly not going to solve every couple's infertility problems, but the approaches you'll read about in Chapters 8 through 12 have been successful in helping many couples get pregnant. Who knows? You just might become the next success story.

Regardless of what type of doctor you work with, be sure to ask the office staff about the cost of office visits and treatment, insurance coverage, and the support resources they offer or to which they can direct you.

STAYING POSITIVE AS YOU TRY TO GET PREGNANT

There are three very important points couples should keep in mind throughout the often-stressful ordeal of infertility, advises Dr. Levine.

- **You're engaged in the ordeal as a couple.** "Your fertility goal is common to you as a couple, and just as a couple shares many ups and downs of life together, so will you share this issue together," says Dr. Levine. "Whether the fertility problem is primarily due to the sperm or to the egg, and whether the fertility treatment itself impacts more on the woman's body or on the man's, the infertility is nobody's 'fault' but is a medical condition to be addressed by you both together as a unit. With this mindset, you as a couple can even draw strength from the ordeal because shared experiences, particularly intensely shared experiences, can bring people closer."

- **You have a medical condition.** "It's just a medical condition," reassures Dr. Levine. "Unfortunately, because reproduction is of such central biologic, social, and religious value, and because most people think of reproduction as such a basic human function that every adult can do it, men and women with fertility problems often feel inadequate as people. Yet people who have problems with their hearts, lungs, or kidneys do not think of themselves as failures; they see their physician, take their medication, and watch their lifestyle. Likewise, people who have problems with their Fallopian tubes or testes should also remember that they have a purely medical problem, and there is no rational basis for feelings of inadequacy or failure."

- **Your condition is treatable.** "Twenty years ago, couples with fertility problems had little hope for medical help, and couples had to resign themselves to the sadness of infertility," notes Dr. Levine. "Now, with modern medicine, this is not the case. For most couples, there is not only hope but the expectation of successful treatment. You do not have to feel that you have been trying to conceive without success, everyone is wondering where's the baby, you are at a loss and do not know what to do, there is no way out. You should not feel this way any more than a person with diabetes should feel trapped by his or her condition. You should seek help, and there is very good help available indeed."

4

When and How
to Conceive

When to conceive is really a multifaceted question. There's the matter of when in your lifetime it's the best to start a family—emotionally, biologically, and financially. Your state of health is also a factor. We've already emphasized how important it is to strive for the healthiest possible body and mind as you focus on trying to get pregnant. For women, knowing when in your cycle you are most fertile is vitally important. Trying to conceive is analogous to jumping rope: getting into the rhythm—the rhythm of your body's cycles—increases your odds of success.

This chapter will help you get to know the ropes. We'll explore some of the pros and cons of having children at various ages and life stages. We'll review the phases of the female reproductive cycle and the accompanying biological changes. You'll learn about how to predict your ovulation each month and how to have sex for the best odds of conceiving. Couples who have already decided that *now* is the time to start a family will find useful information on your journey toward parenthood.

KEEPING TIME: THE BIOLOGICAL CLOCK

A growing number of people are starting families later in life than did earlier generations; yet there's no resetting the biological clock. For women, fertility starts to decline in the late twenties. In fact, the number of eggs that a woman has declines over the years—6 million as a five-month fetus, 2 million at birth, around 400,000 at puberty, and none at menopause—and these eggs are less likely to be fertilized over time. For men, fertility declines with age, especially over the age of fifty, but age is a less dramatic factor than in women. Declining testosterone levels in aging men do cause a modest decline in sperm production and sperm counts, but this doesn't seem to reduce the sperm's ability to fertilize an egg, according to Dr. Zalman Levine, M.D., who was introduced in Chapter 3. He does point out, however, that children born to men over the age of forty have a 20 percent higher chance of having birth defects than children born to younger men.

This doesn't mean that couples in their thirties and forties will necessarily find it difficult to conceive, but it is important to be aware that advancing age can make conceiving and maintaining a pregnancy more of a challenge. The risk of miscarriage increases with age, too. Many women don't realize how much age impacts fertility, according to a recent survey by the American Infertility Association. For couples who are beyond their twenties, the following statistics highlight the importance of doing all you can to increase your odds of conceiving, namely following the healthy habits covered in Chapter 2.

Some Statistics to Consider

- Women are about 30 percent less fertile in their late thirties than they are in their early twenties.

- In a French study, 75 percent of women younger than thirty-one got pregnant within a year of trying. Sixty-two percent of women aged thirty-one to thirty-five got pregnant within a year of trying, and 54 percent of women over thirty-five got pregnant within a year.[1]

- The average time to conception is four to five months for women in their early twenties, five to seven months among women in their late twenties, seven to ten months for women in their early thirties, and ten to twelve months for women in their late thirties.

- High caffeine intake—especially more than 500 mg per day—may delay conception. In a European study reported in the *American Journal of Epidemiology*, in 1997, women with the highest caffeine intake took 11 percent longer to achieve their first pregnancy.[2]

- The risk of miscarriage increases in women aged thirty-five and older; the risk is further increased when the man is also at least forty years old, according to a recent European study.[3]

- The risk of miscarriage is 10 percent at age thirty, 12 percent until age thirty-five, 18 percent in the latter half of the thirties, 34 percent in the early forties, and 53 percent at age forty-five or above, notes Dr. Levine.

- A recent research review found that pregnancy rates were 23 to 38 percent lower in men over age fifty than in men under age thirty when female age was taken into account. The authors concluded that most evidence suggests that higher male age is associated with a decline in sperm motility (movement), semen volume, and sperm morphology (shape), but not with sperm concentration.[4]

Bear in mind that many people have uncomplicated pregnancies and give birth to healthy babies beyond the statistical peak fertility window. And *remember that your chronological age doesn't necessarily correlate with your biological age.* In fact, you can be forty years of age chronologically, yet be either thirty-five or forty-five when it comes to biological age.

You're in charge of your health to a much greater extent than you probably realize, and—depending on your reproductive history—the same applies to your fertility. For example, research has shown that female smokers who continue to smoke close to the time of conception take longer to become pregnant than nonsmokers or women who stop smoking before the year they attempt to conceive.[5] By shedding unhealthy habits and adopting better ones, you and your partner increase your odds of getting pregnant and improve the quality of your life, no matter what your age.

STAGES OF LIFE

Biologically, the early twenties are often considered the ideal years for conception. Fertility is optimal at that life stage, the body can best withstand the stresses of pregnancy, and labor tends to be easier. Staying up all night with babies and running after toddlers is also easier at twenty-two than at, say, thirty-five. Another advantage to starting a family in your twenties is that if you're accustomed to having children from a relatively young age, you don't necessarily know what you're missing in terms of personal time and freedom. Going from a lifestyle without children to one with children later on in life can be a challenging transition.

But there are potential benefits to starting a family a little later. Many people haven't yet attained financial security in their twenties, making the cost of rearing children more of a strain than it might be five or ten years later. Older parents who are more financially secure are more likely to be able to offer their children sport and music lessons and opportunities for other educational experiences. Often they are more established in their careers and, therefore, can devote more energy and time to a family. Older parents also tend to have experienced more of life than those in their twenties. It's likely that they won't have as much desire to stay out late partying as younger people often do, and, generally, they have more life experience (and possibly more patience) to share with their children. On the other hand, among women who are forty and older at the time of conception, there is both an increased risk of chromosomal abnormalities (which can cause Down syndrome and other problems in a developing fetus) and a greater chance that the mother's will experience health problems, such as gestational diabetes and preeclampsia (a toxic condition that may develop in late pregnancy).

Whatever age you are when trying to become pregnant, patience is a virtue. If you have been trying for six months or more and you're a woman under thirty-five, you might want to try the techniques in this book for another six months before consulting a fertility specialist. If you are thirty-five or older and have been trying for at least six months, consider seeing a specialist while following these techniques. There's nothing wrong with bolstering your health and fertility naturally while working with a fertility expert. That's called multitasking. You can be building up your body with healthy habits and formulating a backup plan at the same time.

Collaborative medicine, incorporating the best of all fields, is truly where medicine is headed. Much of the rest of the world uses something other than allopathic medicine, which refers to standard Western medical approaches, as its primary form of health care; natural medicine is the medicine of our ancestors. Yet there are times when conventional medicine is the best or only solution to a health problem. If your appendix is about to rupture, for example, conventional surgery is necessary to take it out. Likewise, some infertility issues require conventional medical procedures in order to resolve them. As in all aspects of life, the key is finding the right balance, in this case among various forms of medicine.

UNDERSTANDING YOUR CYCLE

You may already know the basics about your cycle, but this discussion is intended to help you brush up on your knowledge to improve your odds of getting pregnant. Timing intercourse correctly is incredibly important. According to a survey by the World Congress on Fertility and Sterility, 20 percent of couples seek treatment for infertility unnecessarily; the reason they aren't getting pregnant is because their timing is off.

A typical menstrual cycle, as shown in Figure 4.1, is twenty-eight days, but normal cycles may range from twenty-four to thirty-five days. The first day of menstruation is considered the first day of a new cycle. The cycle is divided into phases: it starts with menstruation (bleeding) and is followed by the proliferative phase (the follicular phase, when the egg/ovum is maturing), ovulation (release of egg), and postovulation (luteal, or secretory, phase).

Menstruation lasts about five days. Tissue fluid, mucus, blood, and epithelial cells from the endometrium (the mucous membrane lining the uterus) make up menstrual flow. Declining levels of estrogen and progesterone (hormones) during this phase cause arteries of the uterus to constrict, leading the cells to die and the *stratum functionalis* layer (the inner layer of the endometrium next to the uterine cavity) to be sloughed off. At this point, the endometrium is at its thinnest. Menstrual flow moves from the uterus to the cervix and out through the vagina.

At the same time, rising levels of follicle-stimulating hormone (FSH) cause pri-

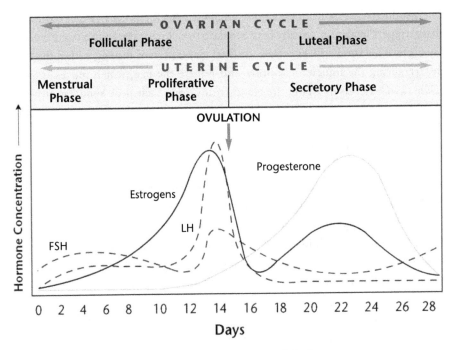

FIGURE 4.1. The Menstrual Cycle

mordial (immature) follicles to develop into primary follicles in the ovaries. Follicles are the fluid-filled sacs that encase eggs in the ovaries. Twenty to twenty-five primary follicles begin to make low levels of estrogen early in each menstrual phase. About twenty of these develop into secondary follicles during the last couple of days in the menstrual phase.

The preovulatory phase takes place after menstruation and before ovulation, and it ranges from six to fourteen days in a twenty-eight-day cycle. One of the twenty or so secondary follicles that start to develop begins to outgrow the others by about day six. The estrogen being secreted by the growing follicles early in this phase cues the body to decrease FSH secretion, so follicles that are not as well developed stop growing. And as the estrogen moves into the bloodstream, it stimulates endometrium growth, doubling its thickness. At the same time, the dominant follicle grows and develops into a mature follicle. At this stage it's ready for ovulation. The egg is microscopic, but the follicles usually grow as large as about 1 inch in diameter right before ovulation. While FSH is the dominant hormone early in the preovulatory phase, luteinizing hormone (LH) increases as ovulation approaches, and right before ovulation the mature follicle produces minimal amounts of progesterone.

A sudden increase in LH caused by high estrogen levels late in the preovulatory phase triggers ovulation, usually between days twelve and sixteen in a twenty-eight-day cycle. This surge of LH causes the final maturation of the egg within the follicle, triggering the follicle to rupture and release the egg, which moves into the pelvic cavity. Levels of LH in the bloodstream reach their peak about twenty-four hours after the LH surge begins, with ovulation occurring about twelve hours after that, or about thirty-six hours after the onset of the LH surge. Levels of LH in the blood and urine are very high during the peak of this surge.

Increasing progesterone levels lead to an increase in basal temperature between 0.4 and 0.6 degrees Fahrenheit, usually about fourteen days into the cycle.

The consistency of cervical mucus provides another cue about when ovulation is occurring. Increased estrogen levels at midcycle cause large amounts of cervical mucus to be produced. This mucus becomes clear and stretchy as ovulation nears. You can monitor this by stretching it between your fingers and noting changes in consistency and degree of stretchiness throughout your cycle. When it stretches the farthest, the time is right.

There are also other clues that ovulation is occurring. For instance, the cervix rises, gets softer, and opens more. Some women have pain in the area of the ovaries. The otherwise acidic pH of the vagina becomes more alkaline, making it more sperm-friendly. To use the jump-roping analogy, you can think of ovulation as the point when the rope hits the ground; it's the ideal time for the sperm to get into the game.

In the postovulatory phase (sometimes referred to as the luteal phase), the mature follicle collapses, turning into a clot that is absorbed by other follicular cells. These cells develop into the corpus luteum, which produces estrogens and progesterone. It's progesterone that gets the uterus (endometrium) ready about a week after ovulation to receive the fertilized egg. With fertilization and implantation, the placenta takes on the hormone-making functions of the corpus luteum. In the meantime, the corpus luteum is maintained by human chorionic gonadotropin (hCG), a hormone made by the chorion. The chorion, or the outer membrane surrounding the fetus that attaches to the uterus, makes the hormone hCG. (That's why hCG is an indicator of pregnancy.) Later the chorion becomes the placenta.

If fertilization and implantation don't happen in a given cycle, LH and gonadotropin-releasing hormone (GnRH) levels decline, and the corpus luteum breaks down and sloughs off. (GnRH stimulates the release of other hormones involved in the cycle.) Levels of estrogen and progesterone drop, leading to the next menstrual phase.

A Success Story

Contributed by Katherine Zieman, N.D.

I had a patient, a young woman in her late twenties, who was not ovulating or having periods on a regular basis. She had not had a complete medical workup of her infertility, as she wanted to start first with simple treatments. I gave her a regimen of herbal medicines to try for six months to promote ovulation and menstruation. She also received a constitutional homeopathic remedy for her general health. After one month she had a regular period, and she conceived at the end of three months.

PREDICTING OVULATION

Over-the-counter home ovulation-predictor kits test for LH in the urine. A positive test signals that LH is surging and that ovulation will happen sometime during the next thirty-six hours. Kits can be used to determine that ovulation will occur in a particular cycle, and they also pinpoint the timing of ovulation. Plus, they're easy to use. You just put a drop of urine on a strip and watch to see if a line on the strip changes color, which indicates that LH is present. Testing can be done daily starting around day ten of your cycle. The vast majority of viable pregnancies are conceived on the day of ovulation and the day preceding it.

Dr. Levine points out that home ovulation-predictor kits are not perfect, however. Daily testing can miss the surge of LH in roughly 20 percent of cycles, he says. Testing both morning and night can improve the accuracy—especially for the 38 percent of women whose LH surge lasts less than ten hours—but the tests will still miss about 10 percent of surges. And an absence of color change on the strip does not necessarily mean that ovulation will not or has not occurred, notes Dr. Levine. He cites a large 1995 study done by the National Institute of Environmental Health Sciences that demonstrates the window of fertility actually begins nearly a week before the LH surge and ends with the day of ovulation.[6] Since the window might end shortly after the surge begins, couples shouldn't wait until the color change to have regular sexual relations for the purpose of conception.

In a test of eleven top-selling ovulation kits, reported in the February 2003 issue of *Consumer Reports*, the ClearPlan Easy Ovulation Test Pack was rated the highest for being easy to read and for its ability to predict ovulation for nearly nine out of ten women. Most women have peak LH surges from less than 20 to 100 mIU/ml (thousandths of an international unit per milliliter), so tests that don't detect LH levels in the lower ranges are not as effective. The ClearPlan Easy Ovulation Test Pack was the only tested product that detected LH concentrations as low as 22 mIU/ml. Twelve percent of women have LH peaks below that concentration, according to *Consumer Reports,* so even the most sensitive test kits will not detect ovulation in these women.

A sister product of the ClearPlan Easy Ovulation Test Pack is a relatively new conception aid called the ClearPlan Easy Fertility Monitor. This product offers the advantage of measuring both levels of estradiol (a form of estrogen), which increase as you near peak fertility around ovulation, as well as LH. The benefit is that it helps identify an extra fertile day early in the window of opportunity. At around $250 ($200 for the monitor and $50 for a pack of thirty replacement urine-test sticks), the palm-sized electronic system is significantly more expensive than other kits, but it also has a memory that stores records for up to six cycles and a digital screen where the optimum time for conception is displayed. In the *Consumer Reports* test, the ClearPlan Easy Fertility Monitor was nearly as sensitive as the ClearPlan Easy Ovulation Test Pack, detecting LH concentrations as low as 36 mIU/ml. These results suggest that it might be useful for about 65 percent of women.

Testing saliva is another method of predicting ovulation. A pattern in dried saliva called *ferning* can be seen under a microscope shortly before ovulation. That kind of testing can also be conducted at home, but the results can be difficult to interpret and, therefore, often unreliable, according to Dr. Levine.

Monitoring and charting changes in basal body temperature, cervical mucus, and other physical signs throughout your cycles can help you estimate your most fertile days. However, Dr. Levine points out that basal body temperature testing can be difficult to interpret and that it retrospectively determines whether ovulation has occurred as opposed to prospectively predicting ovulation. Even so, it may help you get acquainted with patterns in your cycle. Dr. Levine also notes that mucous testing can be cumbersome to perform and difficult to learn, but it is a reliable indicator of imminent ovulation for couples who are motivated to use it.

Homework

Charting Physical Cues to Help Predict Ovulation

Make copies of the chart on pages 72–75 to track these physical cues each month. After a few months, you'll be more familiar with your cycle and will have a better idea of what days to take an LH test to predict ovulation.

To measure basal body temperature, use a basal body thermometer and take your temperature first thing in the morning before getting out of bed. Note the results on a photocopy of the chart in Figure 4.2. Variations throughout your cycle may be subtle and not always consistent from one cycle to the next, but after a few cycles a pattern will emerge. At ovulation you'll observe a dip in temperature followed by a peak.

HOW TO CONCEIVE

As you probably realize by now, timing is a huge factor when you're trying to conceive. "Identifying the days of peak fertility and engaging in sex during those days can go a long way toward helping a couple increase their monthly fertility," says Dr. Levine. So how often should you have sex during the most fertile time in your cycle?

In terms of sperm quality, ejaculating every two or three days is considered ideal. The longer the time between ejaculations, the lower the number of normal, motile sperm in the semen. But repeated ejaculations twenty-four hours or less apart can actually lead to a decrease in the number of sperm. The typically weaker muscle contractions of subsequent orgasms can mean lower sperm count and volume, too. If a man has healthy semen, one orgasm should deliver enough sperm; there's no compelling evidence to suggest that it's necessary to have consecutive orgasms to achieve conception. Sperm motility (the ability to swim through the woman's reproductive system to find the egg) drops when sperm have been stored in the male reproductive tract for more than about seven days, so Dr. Levine suggests that a man should have had an ejaculation within a week prior to trying to conceive during the peak fertility period.

BASAL BODY TEMPERATURE AND MUCUS CHART

Make photocopies of the following pages and fill in the appropriate information.

- To plot your body temperature throughout your cycle, place a dot in the square under the day and across from your temperature. Connect the dots with straight lines.

- In the "Mucus" section, use descriptive words such as creamy, wet, white, clear, sticky, slippery, milky, scant, cloudy, lots, pink, stiff, or translucent based on your observations of your cervical mucus.

- In the "Comments" section, note any circumstances such as fever, illness, travel, stress, lack of sleep, emotional, and so on that may affect your cycle.

BASAL TEMPERATURE AND MUCUS CHART • Month(s) _____

DAY										
DATE										
DAY OF CYCLE	**1**	**2**	**3**	**4**	**5**	**6**	**7**	**8**	**9**	**10**
99.5										
99.4										
99.3										
99.2										
99.1										
99.0										
98.9										
98.8										
98.7										
98.6										
98.5										
98.4										
98.3										
98.2										
98.1										
98.0										
97.9										
97.8										
97.7										
97.6										
97.5										
97.4										
97.3										
97.2										
97.1										
97.0										
Mucus										
Ovulation pain/ pressure										
Comment										

BODY TEMPERATURE

Number of days in this cycle: _____

DAY										
DATE										
DAY OF CYCLE	11	12	13	14	15	16	17	18	19	20

BODY TEMPERATURE

	11	12	13	14	15	16	17	18	19	20
99.5										
99.4										
99.3										
99.2										
99.1										
99.0										
98.9										
98.8										
98.7										
98.6										
98.5										
98.4										
98.3										
98.2										
98.1										
98.0										
97.9										
97.8										
97.7										
97.6										
97.5										
97.4										
97.3										
97.2										
97.1										
97.0										
Mucus										
Ovulation pain/ pressure										
Comment										

Shortest previous cycle: _____

BASAL TEMPERATURE AND MUCUS CHART • Month(s) _____

DAY										
DATE										
DAY OF CYCLE	**21**	**22**	**23**	**24**	**25**	**26**	**27**	**28**	**29**	**30**
99.5										
99.4										
99.3										
99.2										
99.1										
99.0										
98.9										
98.8										
98.7										
98.6										
98.5										
98.4										
98.3										
98.2										
98.1										
98.0										
97.9										
97.8										
97.7										
97.6										
97.5										
97.4										
97.3										
97.2										
97.1										
97.0										
Mucus										
Ovulation pain/ pressure										
Comment										

(Left vertical label: BODY TEMPERATURE)

Number of days in this cycle: _____

DAY										
DATE										
DAY OF CYCLE	31	32	33	34	35	36	37	38	39	40
99.5										
99.4										
99.3										
99.2										
99.1										
99.0										
98.9										
98.8										
98.7										
98.6										
98.5										
98.4										
98.3										
98.2										
98.1										
98.0										
97.9										
97.8										
97.7										
97.6										
97.5										
97.4										
97.3										
97.2										
97.1										
97.0										
Mucus										
Ovulation pain/ pressure										
Comment										

BODY TEMPERATURE

Shortest previous cycle: _____

Having intercourse with ejaculation every forty-eight hours around the time of ovulation is recommended, since healthy sperm can survive about forty-eight hours in the female reproductive tract and the egg is susceptible to fertilization for twelve to twenty-four hours. This conventional recommendation isn't based on firm scientific data, however, cautions Dr. Levine, so it should not be considered an ironclad rule. Daily sex during the fertility window might be the best plan for many couples, he advises. "Although frequent coitus can, indeed, decrease sperm counts," he explains, "this is primarily true only for men whose counts are low to begin with—not for men with normal sperm counts. It's probably reasonable for a couple to have sex as much as they want around the time of ovulation."

There are some additional things you can do to increase your odds of conception when you are most fertile, though not all experts agree on the extent to which they are effective. One common tip is for the woman to put a small pillow under her hips after intercourse for about twenty minutes to keep the cervix in the semen pool, thereby allowing the sperm time to swim up through the cervix. Another way to maximize contact between the cervix and seminal pool is for the woman to lie on her side with her knees bent towards her chest immediately following intercourse. The deepest penetration occurs with the missionary position, so using that might be advantageous because it gets sperm close to the cervix. The same theory explains why some experts suggest positions with the man entering from behind.

Some experts recommend that women avoid straddling their partners during intercourse when trying to conceive because semen can leak out more easily, decreasing the number of sperm that have a chance of making it successfully to the egg. The amount of semen that leaks out following intercourse is probably not enough to greatly impact the odds of conceiving, but if you have trouble conceiving, it's a good idea to try to limit this loss. Depending on sperm counts, this might just make the difference. Avoiding a trip to the bathroom right after sex is another way to keep semen from leaking out. Lying still for fifteen to thirty minutes after sex is probably best.

It's possible that sitting, standing, and women-on-top positions might make it harder for sperm to swim upward against gravity in the woman's reproductive tract. Fortunately, the uterine and vaginal contractions that accompany orgasms help sperm move toward the Fallopian tubes where they attempt to fertilize the egg. For a woman, having an orgasm with semen inside her is likely to help sperm reach their target.

It's important to note that most commercial lubricants sabotage sperm. Unscented mineral oil should be used if lubrication is needed, since it has no adverse effects on sperm, says Dr. Levine. Unscented vitamin E oil is another option. A woman should not douche or rinse out her vagina during the fertility window, as this could wash away viable sperm that survive for about two days in the vaginal canal.

Whatever your sexual style, enjoy yourselves during sex. Trying to get pregnant can be stressful, but don't let yourself get so focused on achieving that goal that you lose sight of the intimacy, compatibility, and attraction to your partner. "Probably the best sex advice for couples interested in fertility is not to focus on fertility, but to maintain the intimacy and emotional intensity of sex," says Dr. Levine. He points to research showing that couples who try to minimize their stress and use relaxation techniques have higher fertility rates both naturally and with assisted reproduction. This makes biological sense, considering the various hormones and chemicals that the body releases during times of relaxation versus times of stress. "It is very important not to let sex become mechanical, a mere form of natural insemination, but to maintain its spontaneity and pleasure," Dr. Levine advises. Relax and enjoy each other. Nature will take its course.

SUMMARY OF TIPS FOR WOMEN

- Chart your basal body temperature, mucus changes, and other physical changes throughout several cycles so you know when you're most fertile.

- Use an LH test kit or an estrogen and LH test kit to target peak fertility in each cycle.

- Optimize the amount of semen inside you during and after intercourse, and strive for orgasms with semen inside you.

- Do not rinse out the vagina at any time during peak fertility.

SUMMARY OF TIPS FOR MEN

- Ejaculate every two or three days for the most potent semen.

- Don't masturbate around the time of ovulation.

- Ejaculate at least once in the week prior to trying to conceive.

SUMMARY OF TIPS FOR MEN AND WOMEN

- Talk to each other about the pros and cons of having children at various ages and make sure you are in agreement about when the time is right to start or continue expanding your family.

- Have sex with orgasms regularly during peak fertility.

- Avoid commercial lubricants, opting for unscented mineral oil or vitamin E oil, as necessary.

- Relax and enjoy the intimacy that you and your partner share.

5

Causes of
Female Infertility

Getting pregnant is a complex process, so it's not surprising that there are several places along the path to conception where there may be obstacles. As noted earlier in the book, about 25 percent of infertility cases are related to a problem with ovarian function and ovulation. Another 25 percent are due to a problem with the woman's Fallopian tubes. Male causes account for at least 25 percent of cases. Seventeen percent of cases are unexplained, and the female disease endometriosis or other assorted causes account for the remainder. Primary infertility is infertility without any previous pregnancy, whereas secondary infertility refers to infertility when there's been a previous pregnancy.

In this chapter, we'll explain the major causes of female infertility and conventional treatments for them. Chapter 6 will cover major causes of male infertility. Some—though not all—of the problems covered in these chapters can sometimes be remedied with natural therapies, which you'll read about in Chapters 8 through 12. Balancing hormones and regulating menstrual cycles, for example, can often be achieved with natural approaches, whereas problems like premature ovarian failure, structural abnormalities, or tubal blockages, which will be discussed here, require conventional medical treatments. Your doctor can help you determine if you are affected by any of these health conditions, and even if testing determines that one of them affects you, it doesn't mean that your odds of getting pregnant and bringing a healthy baby to term are low. If you are affected by one of these conditions, you and your partner can work with your health practitioner to draw up and follow an appropriate plan to enhance your fertility, whether the approach is conventional, natural, or a combination of both.

A CLOSER LOOK AT THE FEMALE REPRODUCTIVE SYSTEM

Before we delve into specific causes of infertility, let's take a look at the female reproductive system. In order to understand the reproductive cycle and how it works, you need to know the parts involved; the success of the parts ensures the success of the whole process of getting pregnant and giving birth.

Virtually the whole female reproductive system is located within the pelvis, as can be seen in Figure 5.1. The entire system is designed to produce a fertile egg from a storage bank of immature eggs, to allow fertilization to occur, and to support the maturation of a baby over about nine months.

External Reproductive Components: The Vulva

The vulva includes all the external tissues that cover the opening to the vagina. These tissues include the mons pubis, hymen, labia, clitoris, and urethra.

- **Mons pubis:** That is the fatty region above the opening to the vagina covered by skin and pubic hair in a sexually mature woman. The mons pubis cushions the pubic region during intercourse.

- **Hymen:** The hymen is a thin fold of mucous membrane that partially covers the vagina. It is normally torn either during the first sexual intercourse or by inserting foreign objects into the vagina.

- **Labia:** There are two pairs of labia, or lips: *labia minora* and *labia majora* (or, simply, smaller lips and larger lips). These surround the opening of the vagina. The labia majora, the outer folds, are covered with hair in a sexually mature woman.

- **Clitoris:** This small mound of erectile tissue and nerves is located toward the top of the vulva, where the folds of the labia come together. It becomes engorged with blood upon arousal and is the counterpart to the male penis.

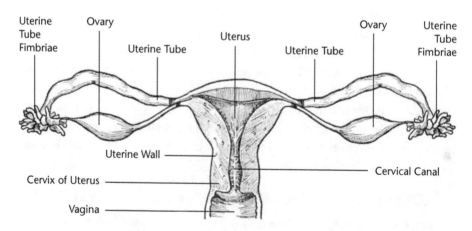

FIGURE 5.1. The Female Reproductive System

- **Urethra:** Situated within the central protected area of the labia, the urethra carries urine from the bladder and is the exit point of the urinary tract. The female urethra is much shorter than the male urethra, which helps explain the higher frequency of urinary tract infection in women; bacteria can gain access to the bladder more readily in women.

Internal Reproductive Components

The vagina, cervix, uterus, Fallopian tubes, and ovaries are interconnected parts of a woman's internal reproductive system.

- **Vagina:** This sex organ, usually about 4 inches long, is a fibromuscular tube that extends from the opening below the urethra to the uterus. Lined with mucous membrane, it is situated between the urinary bladder and the rectum. The vagina receives semen from the penis during sexual intercourse and serves as the passageway for menstrual flow and childbirth. It's also called the "birth canal."

- **Cervix:** Located at the top of the vagina, the cervix is the entrance to and part of the uterus. Cervical mucus typically prevents bacteria, sperm, and other organisms from migrating from the vagina to the uterus, but mucus consistency changes just before ovulation and stays clear and stretchy for a few days to allow sperm to move easily through the uterus to the Fallopian tubes. The cervix stays closed during pregnancy, then it dilates to allow the mature infant to pass through the vagina to the outside world. Physicians examine the cervix and perform Pap tests on it to ensure that the cervix and uterus are healthy.

- **Uterus:** The nonpregnant uterus is about 3 inches long and 2 inches wide. Also called the womb, it is designed to support the developing fetus and is shaped like an upside-down pear. The lining of the uterus builds up each month and then, if pregnancy does not occur, sloughs off in a menstrual period. (For more information on the menstrual cycle, refer to Chapter 4.) When pregnancy does occur, the uterus expands to many times its original size as the developing baby grows within.

The cervical opening, called the "os," allows sperm to enter the uterus. The upper part of the uterus is connected to two Fallopian tubes—one on the right side and one on the left side. Sperm swim through the uterus into the tubes in search of an egg to mate with. If successful, the fertilized egg moves down one tube and into the uterus where it implants itself in the endometrium in the uterine wall. An unfertilized egg is carried away in the menstrual blood.

- **Fallopian tubes:** The Fallopian tubes connect the uterus with the ovaries (glands that contain immature eggs) and serve as the pathway for eggs to reach the uterus. The tubes and their flared ends, or fimbriae, are covered with cilia that catch the egg at ovulation and aid its journey toward the uterus. Fluid and mucus produced in the lining help nourish and move the egg along. The Fallopian tube is the place where egg and sperm unite.

- **Ovaries:** The ovaries are a pair of glands about the size and shape of unshelled almonds. Positioned over each Fallopian tube, an ovary is held in place by ligaments. The ovaries contain all of a woman's ovarian follicles (oocytes, or immature eggs, and their surrounding tissue) at birth. Some of these develop into secondary oocytes and potentially into mature eggs if fertilized. Estrogen, progesterone, inhibin, and relaxin hormones are made in the ovaries.

The Mammary Glands

Mammary glands are the last part of the woman's reproductive system. These modified sweat glands in the breasts are responsible for lactation, which includes producing, secreting, and ejecting milk. The mammary glands are attached to muscles by a layer of connective tissue. Hormones trigger lactation after a baby is born.

THE EGG'S JOURNEY

Let's follow the journey of an immature egg as it prepares for pregnancy. As a female fetus develops, she is creating all the eggs she will ever have, so even before birth the number of eggs a woman will have in her lifetime has already been established. During adolescence when hormones are surging, puberty—the transition from preadolescence to sexual maturation—starts. That's when the young woman begins her menstrual cycle (detailed in Chapter 4), and the process of the monthly maturation of a few eggs begins. The woman is then, if all goes right, capable of becoming pregnant. Changes in secondary sexual characteristics—such as growth of breasts and body hair in the pubic area and under the arms—also occur at puberty.

Every month, one or more eggs released from one of the two ovaries travel down the nearby Fallopian tube. It's important that the tubes are not obstructed by scar tissue from infections or other causes, so the egg can pass through. As the egg travels down a Fallopian tube, changes take place in the uterus to prepare for the arrival of a fertilized egg. Less than 1 percent of the 300 to 500 million sperm cells ejaculated into the vagina reach the secondary oocyte (the form of the egg before fertilization) in the Fallopian tube. Fertilization occurs about twelve to twenty-four hours after ovulation. Right after fertilization, cell division of the fertilized egg, or zygote, begins. This single cell develops into a blastocyst—a hollow ball of cells consisting of an internal cavity, outer cells, and inner cell mass. Once it reaches the uterus, the blastocyst burrows, or implants, into the endometrium that has been prepared for its arrival; this occurs about six days after fertilization. Here is where the baby grows and develops until he or she is ready to greet the world about nine months later. (For a detailed description of the stages of embryonic development, see Chapter 7.)

MAJOR CAUSES OF FEMALE INFERTILITY

Many things contribute to infertility in women, including age, problems with ovulation, blocked or damaged tubes, endometriosis, and miscarriage, among other things. Sometimes the causes of infertility can't be pinpointed, and a diagnosis of unexplained infertility is given.

Age-Related Causes

"Female fertility decreases significantly with advancing age, particularly in the mid-late thirties and forty and older," says Owen K. Davis, M.D., a board-certified reproductive endocrinologist, who is associate director of the Center for Reproductive Medicine and Infertility at the Weill Medical College of Cornell University and president-elect of the Society for Assisted Reproductive Technology (SART). As a woman ages, there are changes in the reproductive hormones that stimulate egg development, cause ovulation, and support a pregnancy. "Even with normal hormonal testing, fertility correlates negatively with age," Dr. Davis points out. All the eggs have been in the ovaries since week eight of fetal development, and they are not replenished. There is a decrease in both the quantity and the quality of eggs with age. The better eggs are released when a woman is younger, explains Shaun C. Williams, M.D., a specialist in infertility and advanced reproductive technology who practices at Pacific Gynecology Specialists in Seattle, Washington. The younger eggs probably have the supporting cells and position in the ovary to respond to lower doses of stimulating hormones. Older eggs are more likely to have hard shells that keep sperm out or genetic defects that keep them from being fertilized or that cause miscarriage.

As a woman ages, more stimulation from the pituitary gland is required to get older eggs to develop. "We see lower pregnancy rates both as a woman ages and as follicle-stimulating hormone (FSH) level rises," Dr. Williams explains. He asserts that women in general are just as fertile today as they were in the past, but our shifting timeline—starting families later in life—highlights the natural effects of aging. A forty-year-old woman has about a 50 percent chance of successful pregnancy, but a forty-five-year-old has less than a 10 percent chance of successful pregnancy, according to Dr. Davis.

Age-related fertility varies among individuals, however, so testing ovarian reserve (the number of good-quality eggs remaining in the ovaries) is important. "An elevated follicle-stimulating hormone (FSH) and/or estradiol level early in the menstrual cycle (around day three) connotes diminished ovarian reserve at any age and is often evaluated early in the fertility evaluation," says Dr. Davis. For this reason, infertility should be evaluated after six months of unprotected intercourse in women over the age of thirty-five and maybe sooner for women forty or older.

Conventional treatment: Aggressive therapy, such as superovulation with fertility medications and intrauterine inseminations, is often undertaken in cases of age-related infertility. In vitro fertilization (IVF) is increasingly used. This procedure unites sperm and egg outside the body in a small, circular dish in a laboratory (not in a test tube, as some people believe); then the fertilized egg is placed in the uterus where it will, hopefully, become implanted in the endometrium. "If the age factor is insurmountable, treatment with donor eggs is highly successful, often exceeding 40 percent," says Dr. Davis.

Ovulatory Disorders

This category includes failure to ovulate (anovulation) or more subtle ovulatory disturbances, such as irregular or long (more than thirty-six days) menstrual cycles. Anovulation is marked by the absence of menstruation or highly irregular menstrual cycles, and diagnosing the underlying cause is a goal in treatment. Polycystic ovary syndrome (PCOS), which often causes male-pattern hair growth, varying degrees of obesity, acne, and insulin resistance, is a common cause of anovulation. Other cases of anovulation stem from disorders of hypothalamic/pituitary function, resulting in inadequate secretion of reproductive hormones. This form of anovulation can be accompanied by weight loss, inadequate body fat, excessive exercise, stress, eating disorders, and disorders of the central nervous system. As with PCOS, doctors try to pinpoint the underlying cause and correct it, if possible.

Another possible ovulatory disorder is luteal phase insufficiency, marked by inadequate progesterone levels in the postovulatory (luteal) phase of the cycle. Luteal phase insufficiency can be diagnosed when there is either low blood progesterone levels or immature endometrial tissue development, which can be determined with an endometrial biopsy, explains Dr. Davis. He notes, however, that there's controversy over whether luteal phase insufficiency is truly a cause of infertility.

Over- or underactive thyroid and elevated prolactin (hyperprolactinemia) should be ruled out through hormone testing and treated if there's a problem. Prolactin is the hormone associated with lactation in women. In men prolactin is associated with prostate growth. Elevated levels in both women and men can lead to infertility.

Conventional treatment: PCOS-related anovulation is typically treated with oral clomiphene citrate, insulin-sensitizing agents (such at metformin), or occasionally, if oral agents are not successful, injectable gonadotropins (substances that stimulate the gonads). Taking clomiphene generally leads to an 80 percent ovulation rate and a pregnancy rate of about 40 percent, according to Dr. Davis. When it's impossible to find and correct the cause of hypothalamic/pituitary dysfunction, injectable gonadotropins are usually successful at inducing ovulation, with monthly success rates around 20 to 25 percent when there are no other infertility factors, notes Dr. Davis. Treatment for luteal phase insufficiency includes progesterone supplementation, clomiphene, and, less commonly, gonadotropins.

Blocked or Damaged Tubes

Fallopian tubes that are blocked or damaged in some way commonly cause infertility by preventing the sperm and egg from uniting naturally. This obstruction or damage can also prevent transport of a fertilized egg into the uterus. Pelvic inflammatory disease (PID), bacteria such as chlamydia, and scarring from pelvic surgery are some common causes of tubal problems. To diagnose this cause of infertility, one of the following is used: laparoscopy, an outpatient surgical procedure in which the pelvis is examined through a small incision in the navel, or hysterosalpingogram, an x-ray of the uterus and tubes after the injection of a special dye through the cervix (for details, see the section "Tests for Couples Who Suspect They Are Infertile" in Chapter 3).

Conventional treatment: Before the advent of IVF, microsurgery was used to open the tubes. Success rates were relatively poor, however, especially when the blockage occurred at the ends of the tubes, according to Dr. Davis. "Blockage where the tube joins the uterus (proximal obstruction) may be effectively treated through cannulation, which entails passing a tube through the cervix to open or widen the tubal opening," he explains. If surgery either is not appropriate or is unsuccessful, IVF—which totally eliminates the role of the tubes—is the most effective treatment. Success rates depend on a woman's age and other factors, but they can exceed 30 to 40 percent. "Whenever tubal disease is diagnosed, IVF should be given serious consideration as first-line therapy," advises Dr. Davis. Tubal surgery is not as commonly performed today as in the past.

A Success Story
Contributed by Katherine Zieman, N.D.

One lovely woman in her early thirties with two children had been try-ing, unsuccessfully, to get pregnant for ten years. She had a long his-tory of endometriosis and chronic PID (pelvic inflammatory disease). Her chronic infection had been treated periodically for years with antibiotics, but it would sometimes reappear, and during this time she never conceived. She sought alternative care because she felt she had exhausted her options in the allopathic medical field. Under naturo-pathic care her chronic infection and endometriosis were treated with herbal medicine, anti-inflammatory supplements, homeopathy, and hydrotherapy. The hydrotherapy consisted of alternating hot and cold sitz baths, which she reported seemed to make the biggest impact on the chronic infection. She ultimately, joyfully, and to her surprise con-ceived and carried a child full-term.

Endometriosis

Endometriosis is a condition in which tissue that normally lines the uterus, called the endometrium, is carried through the tubes, implanting and invading areas within the pelvis, for example, the ovaries. Scarring and distortion of normal anatomy may result. Pelvic pain, painful periods, and pain with intercourse may accompany this condition, though sometimes there are no symptoms.

Conventional treatment: Abnormal tissue can be removed surgically, sometimes relieving symptoms and enhancing fertility, but severe forms may require IVF. Medical treatment of endometriosis with hormones is helpful to alleviate pelvic pain but not to enhance fertility.

Miscarriage

A miscarriage, or spontaneous abortion, is any pregnancy loss that occurs before twenty weeks of gestation (carrying the fetus as it grows in the uterus), or up until about the fifth month. It is often included in the list of infertility causes, since the definition of infertility includes the inability to maintain a pregnancy, in addition to the inability to achieve pregnancy in the first place. Miscarriages can occur very early, sometimes before a woman even knows she's pregnant. They can even be mistaken for a heavy period. Sometimes cramping, passing clots or tissue from the vagina, or bleeding can signify miscarriage. Recurrent miscarriage is commonly defined as three or more consecutive pregnancy losses that occur before fetal viability (fetal weight of 500 grams or twenty weeks gestation).

Fetal and maternal problems are the two major causes of miscarriage. Fetal causes are related to the fetus's genetic makeup. Chromosomal abnormalities, in which the genetic material from egg and sperm don't fuse together correctly, cause about half the miscarriages that occur during the first thirteen weeks. The low percentage of human live births with chromosomal abnormalities suggests that most of these abnormalities are lethal, causing miscarriage early in pregnancy. "The miscarriage is nature's way of discontinuing a terribly abnormal pregnancy," explains Dr. Zalman Levine, M.D. Fetal causes are much more common than maternal causes of spontaneous pregnancy loss. Yet all the scientific rationale for why miscarriages occur cannot take away the confusion, frustration, and sense of loss experienced by women and men who have lost one or more babies to miscarriage.

Maternal causes include factors in the environment where the embryo, and then the fetus, develop. Most of these causes are not related to the conscious activity of the mother or the couple; they include hormonal imbalances (usually due to progesterone), abnormalities in anatomy (usually involving the uterus), serious or life-threatening disease, and immune system problems. Hormonal imbalance can cause miscarriage in women who don't produce enough progesterone because this hormone is needed for the endometrium to nourish the egg properly. Without sufficient progesterone, the egg won't thrive. Maternal illness, including systemic lupus erythematosus, certain heart conditions, uncontrolled high blood pressure, kidney disease, and poorly controlled diabetes might put a woman at higher risk of miscarriage; treating the problem can increase the likelihood of her having a successful pregnancy.

Heavy cigarette smoking, alcohol, or street-drug abuse, medications that are teratogenic (capable of causing malformation of the fetus), and irradiation or exposure to chemical toxins in the workplace, for example, can be causes of miscarriage that are related to the mother's actions. However, miscarriages often occur without being caused by these or any other deleterious actions—conscious or unconscious—on the woman's part. If you are taking medications and are trying to conceive, be sure to ask your doctor if they are considered safe.

Abnormal pregnancies happen more often in older women because of a greater likelihood that an egg will have a chromosomal problem. Keep in mind that eggs sit in the ovary since gestation and are subject to environmental assaults and chromosomal damage over time. This may also mean that there is a tendency for normal eggs to be discharged every month in the early reproductive years, leaving more abnormal eggs for later years, says Dr. Levine. "We know with certainty that the chances of chromosomally abnormal pregnancies, and therefore miscarriages, increase with age," he says. The risk of miscarriage, he notes, is 10 percent until age thirty, 12 percent until age thirty-five, 18 percent in the latter half of the thirties, 34 percent in the early forties, and 53 percent at age forty-five or above.

The good news is that if a woman has a first-trimester miscarriage, she is not at any higher risk of having another miscarriage in her next pregnancy than a woman of her age who has never had a miscarriage. If a woman has two first-trimester miscarriages in a row, however, and if she has had even one second-trimester miscarriage, she should seek consultation from a reproductive endocrinologist, advises Dr. Levine. That's because she or her partner may have an underlying problem that predisposes her to future miscarriages and that can possibly be corrected before future pregnancy attempts.

Conventional treatment: With recurrent pregnancy loss, generally accepted testing, according to Dr. Davis, includes assessment of thyroid function, prolactin (a hormone produce in the brain that is responsible for lactation), evaluation of the luteal phase, evaluation of the uterine cavity (for fibroids, scarring, a congenital septum, or some other problem), and chromosome analysis of the male and female partners. Progesterone deficiency can be diagnosed by monitoring the luteal phase (abnormal if less than twelve days), by low blood progesterone levels, or by immature abnormal endometrial biopsy. "Cervical cultures for potential pathogens are frequently obtained, and in select cases testing for excessive clotting may be appropriate," Dr. Davis says.

After a miscarriage, it is probably best to wait at least six weeks (through a whole normal menstrual cycle) before attempting pregnancy, says Dr. Williams. Though there have been no adverse results reported in women who do get pregnant in the very next cycle, he advises patients to wait.

Couples often blame themselves when miscarriages occur, thinking they must have done something wrong to make it happen. But so often the cause is fetal, not maternal, and is usually beyond the control of either partner. Placing blame on either partner can add guilt to an already intense situation and can make emotional recovery from miscarriage more difficult.

Miscarriages are much more common than most people realize: about one-quarter of all conceptions end in a miscarriage. Even so, that is little comfort for the couple that has lost one or more babies to miscarriage. When dealing with a miscarriage, drawing on your faith and love is important. The loss of a baby, whether full-term or not, is the loss of a baby, and a time of mourning is not unreasonable. Yet it's important to keep a positive outlook and move forward.

The moment a couple finds out that they are pregnant, a bond begins to grow between the unborn baby and parents. Communicating with your partner about the loss of a pregnancy is important, but depending upon that person's coping mechanisms, he or she may or may not be able to communicate their feelings as clearly as you want them to; they may not feel like discussing them at all. Talking with others who have undergone this kind of loss is helpful for some people, while others prefer to mourn privately. Support groups are available to help people deal with their loss and accompanying emotions after a miscarriage, so consider asking the staff at your doctor's office about such resources. (Also, see the Resources section at the back of the book.) Counseling may be helpful in some cases.

The actual process of having a miscarriage can be painful and uncomfortable physically, depending on how far along the pregnancy is and the individual woman's body. Keep in mind that hormones ebb and flow after a miscarriage, much like after a full-term delivery, and they can affect emotions dramatically. Be patient with yourself and your partner. Seek comfort in your faith, if you have one.

Another interesting perspective on miscarriage has to do with destiny. One couple in their early thirties who was interviewed for this book shared their story of having had one child, then getting pregnant again. Around the twelfth week their unborn baby's heart stopped, suggesting that there was a problem with its development. The heartache following that loss caused tremendous stress and challenged their faith. Yet, within four months they were pregnant again, with a child whom they now enjoy completely and who would never have existed if the first pregnancy had gone to term.

Unexplained Infertility

After ruling out the causes of infertility described above, as well as male factors (discussed in Chapter 6), a diagnosis of unexplained infertility is made.

Conventional treatment: "Treatment depends on the female partner's age (more aggressive if she's older) and may include intrauterine inseminations with or without fertility drugs (clomiphene, gonadotropins) and IVF," says Dr. Davis.

Other Causes of Infertility

"The infertility evaluation has historically included other tests, such as the post-coital test, to assess the interaction of the sperm with the cervical mucus ('cervical factor')," says Dr. Davis. Yet studies have shown that this test is generally unreli-

A Success Story

Contributed by Katherine Zieman, N.D.

A sad and frustrated couple came to me because of the woman's inability to carry a pregnancy past the first trimester. The woman was in her late twenties and had a history of seven miscarriages. When she conceived for the eighth time, she started on a regimen of herbal medicines to both prevent miscarriage and promote uterine tone by balancing her hormones. Finally and ecstatically she was able to carry a child to full-term. She has since delivered four more children and has found that she can prevent miscarriage as long as she takes the herbal medicine from conception until the end of the first trimester.

able. Cervical factor is a relatively uncommon cause of infertility, probably accounting for less than 5 percent of cases, according to Dr. Davis. Evaluating male and female patients for antisperm antibodies (called "immunologic factor") can be useful in select cases, but this isn't part of the basic infertility evaluation. Screening for infectious agents, such as bacteria like chlamydia and others, is often done, but cause and effect when there is no tubal factor is controversial. Even so, this kind of testing is probably reasonable, says Dr. Davis, since it's relatively simple and eradicating potentially harmful bacteria is prudent. Routine testing for autoimmune disorders or clotting abnormalities is not supported by current practice, except when the couple's history calls for it. Some examples would be recurrent second- or third-trimester pregnancy losses, otherwise unexplained clotting problems, and venous thrombosis, a condition in which there's a blood clot in a deep vein, usually in the lower leg or thigh.

DEBUNKING INFERTILITY MYTHS

By now you should have a sense of where things can go wrong in the complex process of conception, at least on the female side of things. Our hope is that this information will empower you and your partner as you strive to boost your fertility, get pregnant, and eventually give birth to a healthy, happy baby. This is also our intent with Chapter 6, in which you'll read about male causes of infertility. The more you know about potential obstacles to conception, the better prepared you'll be to deal with any fertility challenges you may face.

According to Dr. Levine, some infertility myths need to be debunked. While we encourage readers to pursue natural options to overcoming infertility whenever possible, some cases require assisted reproductive technologies such as IVF, discussed by Dr. Levine below. You can learn more about this procedure and others from resources listed at the back of the book.

- **Until I've tried for a year to get pregnant, no one will take me seriously if I ask for help.** "When you should seek help depends on your situation," says Dr. Levine. "If you are a woman thirty-five or older, you should seek help after at most six months of unsuccessful attempts, perhaps three months if you are forty or older. If you are a woman of any age and have menstrual cycles that are irregular—even somewhat irregular—you should seek input earlier rather than later. If you as a couple are having sexual difficulties that are not improving, you should seek advice without waiting at all. Better to seek medical help and find out you don't really need it than to need help and not seek it."

- **Fertility treatment can cause me to have septuplets like that woman in Iowa.** "It's certainly true that the problem of multiple pregnancy with assisted reproduction has been an escalating one," says Dr. Levine. "Recent data from the year 2000 have shown that from 1980 to 2000, the number of twin births in the U.S. increased by over 50 percent and the number of high-order multiple births (triplets or more) increased almost fivefold. Assisted reproduction is admittedly one of the major causes of this rise. However, with close monitoring in the hands of your physician, and with everyone's understanding that your fertility treatment must be modified or even cancelled if the risk of multiple pregnancy looks like it's becoming too high, this is a controllable problem and the risk to you can be kept very much to a minimum."

- **I am scared of IVF. It's like science fiction and seems scary and experimental.** "IVF in 2004 is far from science fiction," reassures Dr. Levine. "The first IVF baby was born in 1978, so the technology has existed now for [more than] twenty-five years. It is also far from experimental; IVF is performed in hundreds of centers throughout the world. Several hundred thousand IVF babies have been born in the United States alone. It's normal for IVF to sound scary to you as a couple. Most fertility offices well understand this and provide a lot of personalized support for you to educate you about the process and to guide you as you undergo it. IVF has become an important part of our clinical armamentarium, allowing us, with success undreamed of even fifteen years ago, to help couples who would otherwise have had no medical hope. If you need IVF, do not fear it. Learn about it, find support with others going through it, and hopefully celebrate your success from it."

- **I need IVF and want to go to the center with the highest published success rates.** "The Society for Assisted Reproductive Technology, in conjunction with the Center[s] for Disease Control, publishes an annual report of IVF success rates for every accredited center in the United States," notes Dr. Levine. "However, these numbers can be very misleading, and it is very difficult to compare centers based on these numbers alone. For one thing, the published numbers lag by approximately two years, so they do not provide recent information on the workings of the center. Also, some centers may unfortunately be overly concerned with the appearance of their published numbers to the extent that, in order to maintain their statistics, they may deny care to couples who might not have the highest chance of success. Be wary of this, and understand that most accredited IVF centers will provide you with similar chances of success from IVF. The most important factor is to find a physician you are comfortable with and a center that will give you personalized, professional, and compassionate care."

6

Causes of
Male Infertility

Male factors account for up to a third of infertility cases, and there are a wide variety of causes. Sperm quantity and quality, varicose veins around the testicles (varicocele), and obstruction are among the conditions that can hinder male fertility. We'll describe them and the conventional treatments for them in the following pages.

When it comes to enhancing your fertility, knowledge is power. The research on natural therapies that can enhance fertility is strong, yet most of the available statistics on success rates refer only to conventional approaches. As you read about male fertility challenges, remember that the information about natural therapies in Chapters 8 through 12 is provided to help you overcome some of them.

Let's begin by coming to grips with the nature of the challenge, so that we can build the best strategies to improve your odds of victory. First, we'll take a look at the male reproductive system; understanding how things work can help us cope with any malfunction. After all, that's how we fix things around the house or at work; it all starts with understanding the parts and how they work together.

A CLOSER LOOK AT THE MALE REPRODUCTIVE SYSTEM

The male reproductive system is designed for sexual intercourse and for fertilization of the ova (eggs) with sperm. Much of the male reproductive tract is outside the body, but important components are housed within the pelvis. During adolescence mature sperm begin to be produced. At the same time, the effects of testosterone deepen the voice of a young male and cause the growth of facial, armpit, and pubic hair. Before reviewing the journey the sperm take on their way to leaving the body, let's take inventory of the various male reproductive parts. (Refer to Figure 6.1.)

- **Testicles:** The two testicles, or testes, are made up of a series of conduits that allow sperm to traverse the duct system, including the *epididymis* and *vas deferens*. The oval-shaped testicles become 1 to $1\frac{1}{2}$ inches long when fully mature.

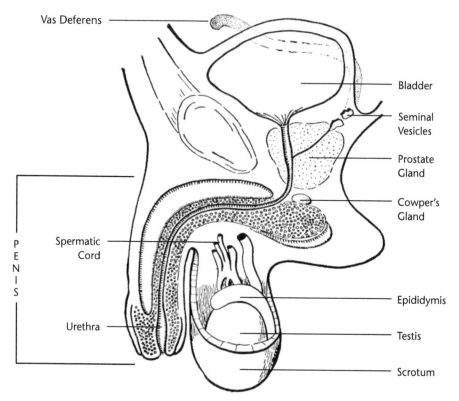

FIGURE 6.1. The Male Reproductive System

They produce and store tiny sperm cells that give rise to mature sperm. They also produce testosterone, often called the male hormone, though women produce low levels of testosterone, too. The testicles are the counterpart of the female ovaries.

- **Tubules:** The seminiferous tubules and straight tubules are located in the testes and carry sperm to the epididymis, which houses the ductus epididymis, where sperm mature.

- **Scrotum:** This pouchlike sac contains the testes (the organs that produce sperm). The scrotum maintains the testes' temperature at about two degrees C below the temperature of the internal organs, which enables sperm to be created. The cremasteric muscles help maintain this temperature by dropping the testes away from the body when scrotal temperature is too high and pulling the testes closer to the body when they get too cold.

- **Epididymis:** One of two organs shaped like commas and located along the posterior borders of the testes. Sperm mature fully in the ductus epididymis after which they are transported to the vas deferens.

- **Vas deferens:** These muscular tubes pass upward along the testes into the lower pelvis and transport the sperm-containing fluid, called semen, to the ejaculatory ducts.

- **Penis:** The male sex organ consists mostly of erectile tissue, the urethra, blood vessels, and surrounding skin. The penis becomes erect when aroused and makes possible intercourse and delivery of sperm to the vagina. It's divided into the shaft and the head, or glans penis, which is the most important source of nerve impulses that signal sexual response. The penis becomes erect when the arteries within it become dilated and the erectile tissue fills with blood (more blood flows into the tissue than out). A membrane made of hard fibers significantly increases the pressure within the expanding erectile tissue, rendering the penis hard and elongated.

- **Urethra:** The tube that carries urine and, during sexual arousal, semen through the penis.

Accessory Glands

The accessory glands provide the lubricant that oils the ducts and nourishes the sperm. They include the seminal vesicles, the prostate gland, and the Cowper's glands.

- **Seminal vesicles:** These saclike, paired glands are attached to the vas deferens along the side of the bladder and produce seminal fluid and fructose, a sugar that fuels the sperm's journey to the egg.

- **Prostate gland:** Located inside the body, the prostate gland produces some of the components of semen. It surrounds the neck of the bladder and is located just at the base of it. This explains why, when the prostate gland swells (as it normally does with aging), men have difficulty urinating. This is the gland your physician feels when he or she inserts a finger into the rectum.

- **Cowper's glands:** These glands, also called bulbourethral glands, lie on either side of the urethra at the base of the penile shaft and add a small amount of lubricant to semen before ejaculation occurs.

THE SPERM'S JOURNEY

Let's follow the sperm's journey through the male reproductive system. While women are born with all the eggs they will have in a lifetime, mature males are constantly producing new sperm. Sperm—or spermatozoa, as mature sperm cells are scientifically called—normally mature at a rate of about 300 million per day. Cell division produces spermatozoa that contain 50 percent of a man's genetic code. Each sperm-producing cycle consists of six stages and takes about sixteen days to complete. Approximately five cycles, or two-and-a-half months, are needed to produce one mature sperm. As a result, changes in your diet, lifestyle, and other therapies may take a few months to show up in lab tests. Sperm development is ultimately controlled by the endocrine (hormonal) system.

Shaped like tiny tadpoles, sperm are designed to reach and penetrate a female ovum, or egg. Each sperm has a head, midpiece, and tail. The head contains the nuclear material and the *acrosome*, a dense granule containing enzymes that help the sperm penetrate an ovum (also called a secondary oocyte). Mitochondria (cell structures often referred to as the "powerhouses" of cells) in the sperm's midpiece are responsible for metabolism, which provides energy for locomotion. The tail propels the sperm forward on its journey. After ejaculation, sperm have a life expectancy of about forty-eight hours inside the female reproductive tract.

The sperm begin their journey within the testes in the seminiferous tubules that lead to other tubules called straight tubules, then move to the epididymis and on to the vas deferens and then the urethra. During an orgasm in intercourse, sperm are ejaculated from the penis and begin their trip inside the woman's reproductive tract by swimming up the vagina toward the egg. Sperm travel in a fluid called semen, a mixture of sperm and secretions of the seminal vesicles, Cowper's glands, and prostate gland. Not only does semen transport and nourish sperm, it neutralizes the acidic environments of the male urethra and female vagina so both become more sperm friendly. This mixture of sperm and secretions also contains enzymes that activate sperm after they are ejaculated, and it contains an antibiotic called *seminal plasmin* that can destroy certain bacteria in semen and the female reproductive tract that have the potential to hinder fertilization. The average volume of semen per ejaculation is 2.5 to 5 milliliters, with 50 to 150 million sperm per milliliter. (Sperm levels below 20 million/milliliter tend to result in infertility.) A very tiny percentage of these sperm eventually reach the ovum, so a large number is required to increase the odds. Only one sperm is actually needed to fertilize an egg, but additional sperm are required to help out at the egg. They are needed to secrete substances from the acrosomes that digest the barrier material surrounding the egg so a single sperm can penetrate it. (See Chapter 7 for details on the development of the embryo once the egg has been fertilized.)

MAJOR CAUSES OF MALE INFERTILITY

Now you know how the male reproductive equipment normally works. Here's a look at some of the problems that can prevent fertility when some part of the system is not functioning properly.

Varicocele

Varicocele, a condition marked by a number of dilated veins around the testicles, is the most common abnormality found during a male infertility evaluation and the most common correctable cause of male infertility. Varicocele is responsible for 42.2 percent of male infertility,[1] but not all men who have a varicocele are rendered infertile; about 15 percent of fertile men also have this condition. Most varicoceles occur on the left side, but as many as 20 percent occur on both sides, according to Peter N. Kolettis, M.D., assistant professor of medicine at the University of Alabama at Birmingham and a specialist in male infertility. Varicoceles may impair sperm production by raising scrotal temperature, but it's not clear exactly how they cause infertility.

Conventional treatment: Surgical and nonsurgical procedures can correct varicocele on an outpatient basis, with equivalent success rates, says Dr. Kolettis. During the procedure, the dilated veins are blocked off (occluded) to allow blood to flow through normal veins instead. After the procedure roughly two-thirds of men show improved semen analysis, and about 40 percent are able to initiate a pregnancy.[2] Improvements aren't seen until at least three months after correction.

Dr. Kolettis points out that there is some controversy about whether these procedures are truly beneficial. Most studies on varicoceles have been uncontrolled, making it difficult to interpret results. For example, a man who impregnates his spouse following varicocele correction might have contributed to a pregnancy without it. Two controlled studies, however, found improvement in semen analysis with correction, and one of these studies demonstrated increased odds of pregnancy following correction.[3,4]

Obstruction

Obstruction, or blockage, is the second most common correctable cause of infertility, accounting for 14.3 percent of cases. It is most often a result of vasectomy, male surgical sterilization where a part of each vas deferens is cut and removed, so that sperm is no longer carried in semen during ejaculation. Sometimes the epididymis, which is the site of sperm maturation, becomes blocked later, as well.

Conventional treatment: About 6 percent of men who have vasectomies request a reversal, which can be performed on an outpatient basis with local or general anesthesia. The odds of sperm returning to the semen depend on the amount of time that has passed since the vasectomy, the appearance of fluid from the vas deferens,

Debunking Infertility Myths
Contributed by Philip Werthman, M.D.

Philip Werthman, M.D., is chief of urology at Century City Hospital in Los Angeles and an expert on male reproductive health. For more information about him, including the Sperm Chromatin Structure Assay (SCSA), which he administers to test for sperm DNA damage, visit www.malereproduction.com.

- **If a couple is infertile, it must be the woman's fault.** "Infertility is truly a couples' issue where a male factor contributes in almost half the cases," says Dr. Werthman. "Both the female and male partners need to be examined and tested when a couple fails to conceive within a year of trying."

- **Taking testosterone improves sperm counts.** "Testosterone is needed for sperm production," notes Dr. Werthman, "but when testosterone supplements are taken they actually stop the testicles from producing sperm by shutting down the normal hormonal signals from the brain to the testicles. This leads to temporary and sometimes permanent sterilization. Men who are interested in becoming fathers should not take testosterone."

- **Men with abnormal sperm counts don't need to see a doctor.** "An abnormal sperm count could be the sign of a serious health problem such as testicular cancer, hormone imbalance, genital infection, thyroid or genetic problem," asserts Dr. Werthman. "All men with an abnormal semen analysis should be evaluated by a specialist in the field of male infertility."

- **The treatment for male infertility is in vitro fertilization.** "Since its inception in the mid-1990s, IVF has enabled many men with very low sperm counts to become biological fathers," states Dr. Werthman. "Unfortunately, the technology designed to help the worst and most refractory cases of male infertility is being applied to all men across the board when the sperm count isn't completely normal. This push to IVF has been driven by some of the doctors who perform IVF and by the pharmaceutical companies that manufacture the expensive drugs used during an IVF cycle. Men with an abnormal semen analysis must be examined to try and find the cause of the problem and make sure it is not a serious condition. Many causes of male infertility can be treated very cost effectively and IVF can be avoided."

- **Vasectomy reversal doesn't work (men stop producing sperm after a vasectomy).** "This is a common misconception that I have heard told to patients by both gynecologists and urologists who don't perform many vasectomy reversals," clarifies Dr. Werthman. "This is based on the old studies of vasectomy reversals prior to the refinement of the vasoepididymostomy surgery. Back then all patients who had a vasectomy reversal underwent a vasovasostomy even if they had a second blockage in the epididymis. Obviously a vasovasostomy will fail in that situation. Success rates for older vasectomies have increased dramatically with the advent of the refined vasoepididymostomy and new microsurgical techniques. The latest study to look at success rates of vasectomy reversal performed fifteen years or more after vasectomy shows that the pregnancy rates for intervals of fifteen to nineteen years, twenty to twenty-five years, and greater than twenty-five years are 49 percent, 39 percent, and 25 percent, respectively."

• **All you need is a few live sperm in order to have a baby with IVF.** "While this was the belief among infertility specialists until recently, it is now clear that the quality of the sperm is an important factor in conception and delivering a healthy baby," asserts Dr. Werthman. "New tests have been developed to analyze the DNA integrity of the sperm. If there is a high level of damage, then the chance of conception is poor no matter what technology is used to fertilize the egg. Damage to sperm can be corrected in many instances."

• **Men who are trying to conceive should wear boxer shorts and not briefs.** "While heat is really bad for sperm," notes Dr. Werthman, "several studies show no difference in sperm quality when the men wore either boxers or briefs. Jacuzzi tubs and hot baths should be avoided."

whether or not there is a secondary obstruction in the epididymis, and surgical experience and technique, says Dr. Kolettis. Pregnancy rate after reversal depends on these factors, in addition to the female partner's fertility. In the largest study of vasectomy reversals, examining the results of more than 1,400 microsurgical procedures, the chances for success decreased as the time since vasectomy increased.[5] (See Table 6.1 on page 100.)

The longer the time since the vasectomy, the greater the chance there will be obstruction of the epididymis. If that's the case, a vasovasostomy (a procedure reconnecting the two ends of the vas deferens) won't be successful, Dr. Kolettis explains. Instead, a vasoepididymostomy (a procedure connecting the vas deferens to the epididymis, thereby bypassing the obstruction) is necessary. "Vasoepididy-

TABLE 6.1. POTENCY AND PREGNANCY RATES AFTER VASECTOMY REVERSALS

TIME SINCE VASECTOMY	POTENCY RATE*	PREGNANCY RATE
[less than] 3 years	97 percent	76 percent
3–8 years	88 percent	53 percent
9–14 years	79 percent	44 percent
15 years or more	71 percent	30 percent

percent chance of sperm returning to semen

mostomy is a significantly more complex and time-consuming procedure," notes Dr. Kolettis. "With this procedure, however, improved success rates can be achieved for cases where a long time has lapsed since the vasectomy." The following results from a very recent study illustrate this point.[6] (See Table 6.2.)

TABLE 6.2. PREGNANCY RATES IMPROVE WITH VASOEPIDIDYMOSTOMY

TIME SINCE VASECTOMY	PREGNANCY RATE
15–19 years	49 percent
20–24 years	39 percent
25 years or more	25 percent

Poor Sperm Quality, Quantity, and Morphology

Infections, high fevers, genetic conditions, and lifestyle factors (Jacuzzi use and smoking, for example) are some causes of poor sperm quality. It's important to remember that your sperm represents your genetic code. The communication of the message encoded in your sperm must be of high quality, as well as precise and accurate. The best way to help ensure high-quality sperm is to nourish your body well—which you read about in Chapter 2 and will read more about in Chapter 8. The next best way is to lessen the burdens that can compromise your health or zap your nutritional stores. Steering clear of environmental toxins, which we covered in Chapter 2, is another way to protect sperm quality. Even men with normal sperm counts may be infertile if the majority of their sperm are nonmotile (don't move well) or abnormally shaped. Morphology refers to their shape; normally shaped sperm are desired for optimal fertility. "Normal" sperm values are from 1.5 to 5 milliliters of volume (semen per ejaculate), with a density of at least 20 million sperm per milliliter, of which more than 30 percent are motile (able to move) and more than 60 percent are normal in shape.

Sperm quality does decline with age, but it varies based on the individual. "We start seeing a decline in the forties, but there are clearly men in their eighties who father children," says Dr. Werthman. "If a man is having difficulty conceiving, he should be evaluated to make sure he doesn't have a serious condition such as testicular cancer or pituitary/endocrine problems. Men with abnormal sperm should be evaluated and treated, not just shoved into IVF. I have seen too many couples spend tens of thousands of dollars doing in vitro without success because of poor sperm quality and the man was never sent for an evaluation to diagnose and improve the problem." DNA damage to sperm can hinder fertility significantly, and tests can determine the health of sperm.

There is a strong correlation between fertility and the number of sperm in an ejaculation. Deficient sperm production causes about 90 percent of cases of low sperm count.[7] In the vast majority of cases, the cause of decreased sperm formation is not known, and the condition is labeled *idiopathic oligospermia* for unexplained low sperm count (under 5 to 10 million per milliliter of ejaculate) or *azoospermia* if no living sperm are found in semen. According to the Center for Male Reproductive Medicine (www.malereproduction.com), nearly 20 percent of men with azoospermia or severe oligospermia have an identifiable genetic cause of infertility. A specialist in male fertility can address this problem.

Conventional treatment: Unfortunately, there is very little that the conventional model has to offer to improve sperm counts. If they are due to elevated levels of prolactin (a hormone involved in prostrate growth), avoiding drinking alcohol is very important, and taking the drug bromocriptine can help lower prolactin levels, thus helping improve sperm production. Likewise, if testosterone levels are low, supplemental medication to increase the levels can be helpful. If excess estrogen is present, the chemotherapy drug tamoxifen (Nolvadex), which possesses anti-estrogenic properties, can help stimulate the release of gonadotropin (a hormone that stimulates the gonads), which will, in turn, lead to sperm production. Also, tremendous advances have been made with in vitro fertilization, which you can read more about in books listed in the References section at the back of the book. When a sperm and an egg are united in a laboratory dish, as in IVF, the number of sperm a man produces becomes less of a factor.

Ejaculatory Dysfunction

This category includes premature ejaculation, ejaculating too soon during sex, and retrograde ejaculation, when semen is ejaculated into the man's bladder rather than out through the penis. Sometimes all, or sometimes only a portion, of the semen enters the bladder, with the rest leaving the penis normally.

A Success Story

Contributed by Richard, age 47, with Olivia, age 33

Like lots of couples, we decided we wanted to have a baby and started trying, but nothing happened. Then Olivia thought she would have to figure out more about her basal body temperature and when she was fertile, but still nothing happened. I suppose each of us thought, "It's probably me." So we each went to a doctor. Olivia went to her obstetrician/gynecologist, who looked at her charts and said everything looked pretty good. She also went to a nutrition lecture by a naturopathic doctor, since that was something she was interested in. My general practitioner said, "You've got to try to do timing." I said we had been doing that. Then he said, "We can do a sperm test." Two things came from it. My doctor said, "Your sperm count is low. I want you to go to a urologist." At the end of the visit with the urologist, he said, "Everything looks fine." But I said, "Actually, this is a fertility thing." Then he looked at the report and said, "Well, you should be thinking about adoption." When I told Olivia, she said, "I'm going to call the naturopath and make an appointment." She explained the issues and that person recommended we see Susan Roberts [a practicing N.D. in Portland, Oregon]. When Olivia explained what was going on, Susan Roberts said that even though she mostly dealt with female patients, we could give it a shot. She did a CBC test [a complete blood count, detailed in Chapter 3], and it ended up that I was really, really anemic. She gave me dietary supplements—zinc, arginine, coenzyme Q_{10}, B_{12}, iron, vitamin C, and carnitine. I noticed that almost all the dietary supplements were things I'd seen on lists of precursors to sperm production. I also took an herbal tincture twice a day. We called it the "stinkture" because it smelled awful. By the end of the second month, I didn't need a refill because Olivia was pregnant. Our son is a year and a half now, and I guess I'm going to have to start taking the stinkture again because we want to have another baby.

Conventional treatment: Premature ejaculation is much more common than most people realize. However, it's not something that men discuss freely, certainly not in locker rooms. Premature ejaculation when the penis is within the vagina will not interfere with fertility. Problems arise if the man ejaculates before entering the woman, though some women have been known to become pregnant when ejaculate is outside the vagina.

Premature ejaculation can be treated with mental conditioning that desensitizes a man who becomes overexcited. Or a physician can prescribe creams that numb the penis to stimulation. If there are underlying health issues, such as anxiety or other conditions, the appropriate medication is important.

Men with retrograde ejaculation are sometimes counseled to take sodium bicarbonate the day prior to intercourse to make the urine more alkaline, since sperm are more likely to survive in an alkaline environment.

Disorders of Accessory Glands and Immunity

This category includes such things as infection, inflammation, and antisperm antibodies. In some men (and women), the immune system mistakes sperm for foreign substances and creates antisperm antibodies that destroy the "invading" cells. The antibodies attach themselves to sperm and hinder their ability to fertilize an egg.

Conventional treatment: Treatment varies based on the specific problem, which a fertility expert can help identify and treat accordingly. Steroids are sometimes prescribed to destroy antibodies that hinder sperm. Another approach is washing sperm that has been collected (after masturbation) to remove antibodies. The sperm can then be injected into the woman via intrauterine insemination (IUI) or into a lab dish that contains eggs retrieved from the woman during IVF.

Coital Disorders

This category includes premature withdrawal, technique problems, and erectile dysfunction.

Conventional treatment: Premature withdrawal is simply remedied by coaching the man to prolong intercourse until ejaculation occurs. Technique problems can generally be eliminated by keeping sex simple, such as using the missionary position. It's not advisable to have sex when standing, if technique is a concern. Also, encourage your partner to remain lying down after sex for twenty to thirty minutes without getting up to urinate; this might help make the difference.

With the advent of Viagra and other such medications, erectile dysfunction has become easier to treat. Still, numerous health issues, such as diabetes, and drugs can cause erectile dysfunction (see "Some Causes of Erectile Dysfunction"). It is worth noting that research has shown that some men, after discussing it with their physician, may benefit from taking the herb ginkgo biloba if they take selective serotonin

Some Causes of Erectile Dysfunction

- Atherosclerosis
- Pelvic surgery and trauma
- Use of the following drugs:
  - Antidepressants
  - Antihistamines
  - Antihypertensives (taken for high blood pressure)
  - Antipsychotics
  - Sedatives
- Alcohol and tobacco
- Diabetes

- Low thyroid
- Decreased male hormones
- Elevated prolactin levels
- Increased serum estrogen
- Prostate disorders
- Neurological conditions:
  - Multiple sclerosis
  - Spinal nerve impingement
- Psychological causes
- Stress

reuptake inhibitor (SSRI) antidepressants. (For more information on natural ways to treat erectile dysfunction, see *Better Sex Naturally* by Chris D. Meletis, Harper-Collins, 1999.)

WEIGHING YOUR OPTIONS

This chapter covers the most common causes of male infertility. If you and your doctor determine that you are affected by these or possibly other causes, it's time to weigh your treatment options. Sometimes conventional methods are the best (and sometimes the only) way to correct the problem. In many cases, however, natural medicine offers help and hope. In Chapters 8 through 12 you and your partner will learn more about these natural strategies for overcoming infertility. But before that, let's take a look at what happens when the male and female reproductive systems work normally and harmoniously to unite the sperm and egg that eventually leads to the birth of a healthy baby. Hopefully, you will soon be witnessing the magic of this union in your own lives.

7

Conception:
The Beginning of a Miracle

When the male and female reproductive systems are working well and the timing is right, the wondrous process of creating a new life takes place. Now it's time to visualize success. In this chapter we'll take a look at the stages of an embryo's development from the time that sperm and egg come together to form the new life. Gestation refers to the amount of time a zygote, embryo, or fetus is carried in the female reproductive tract.

CONCEPTION TO BIRTH: A MIRACULOUS
AND AWE-INSPIRING JOURNEY

During intercourse sperm enter the vagina and swim through the opening in the cervix, the os, which is the gateway to the uterus. The sperm swim toward the top of the uterus, which connects to the Fallopian tubes. Less than 1 percent of the 3 to 5 million sperm cells ejaculated into the vagina actually reach the egg. The sperm are helped along by an enzyme called *acrosin,* produced by the acrosome in the sperm, that stimulates motility and migration in the female reproductive tract. Prostaglandins, created by the woman's body in reaction to semen, stimulate muscular contractions of the uterus. It is thought that these chemicals work in the uterus to propel sperm toward the unfertilized egg, and the egg is thought to secrete a chemical substance to attract sperm, as well. Sperm aren't capable of fertilizing an egg until they have spent about ten hours in the female reproductive tract. The tract actually helps make sperm capable of fertilizing an egg; the changes sperm undergo here are called *capacitation.* The membrane around the acrosome becomes fragile, and the acrosome begins to secrete destructive enzymes. These enzymes help penetrate the layers of follicular cells around the egg, which are called the *corona radiata* and the *zona pellucida;* the corona radiata are cells that surround and protect the zona pellucida, while the zona pellucida is a gelatinous layer where sperm attach. Normally, one spermatozoon penetrates and enters an egg, an event called *syngamy.*

A series of events that follow prevent polyspermy, or fertilization by more than one spermatozoon. At this point, the egg (secondary oocyte) begins dividing into a larger ovum (mature egg) and a smaller part that fragments and disintegrates. Fertilization usually takes place in a Fallopian tube about twelve to twenty-four hours after ovulation.

Once the sperm has entered the egg, it sheds its tail, and the nucleus in its head becomes a structure called the male pronucleus. The nucleus of the egg becomes a female pronucleus; then the two fuse, resulting in a segmentation nucleus containing twenty-three chromosomes from the male pronucleus and twenty-three from the female pronucleus. The fertilized egg, now called a zygote, consists of cytoplasm, a segmentation nucleus, and zona pellucida. There is some debate about when conception actually occurs. Most believe it's when the sperm penetrates the egg, while others believe it occurs once fusion takes place. At the moment of conception, the zygote is about the size of a grain of sand. When two eggs are released and each is fertilized by different spermatozoa, dizygotic (fraternal) twins result. Each is genetically unique and can be either gender. Monozygotic (identical) twins develop when a single fertilized egg splits at an early stage of development. Monozygotic twins have exactly the same genetic material and are always the same sex.

Here's an overview of what happens after the egg is fertilized: The first two months are considered the embryonic period, and the developing human is called an embryo. The fetal period refers to the months of development after the second month, and the developing human is called a fetus. In the discussion below, we often refer to both embryo and fetus as "your baby."

Day 1 to Day 4

During the first day after fertilization, the zygote begins to divide by multiples of two. One becomes two, then two become four, four become eight, and so on. The first of the rapid cell divisions, called cleavage, is completed about thirty-six hours after fertilization. The rest of the divisions take a bit less time, with the second cleavage completed by the second day after fertilization. There are sixteen cells by the end of the third day. The solid mass of cells, still surrounded by zona pellucida and referred to as the *morula,* remains about the same size as the original zygote. The number of cells in the morula increases and keeps moving along the Fallopian tube toward the uterus by the end of the fourth day. The cluster of cells develops into a hollow ball of cells called a blastocyst, which enters the uterus at four-and-a-half to five days. A part of the blastocyst later forms part of the fetal portion of the placenta, and the inner-cell mass becomes the embryo.

Day 5 to Day 9

The zona pellucida disintegrates when the blastocyst is in the uterus but before the blastocyst attaches to the uterine lining (endometrium). Secretions from the endometrial glands nourish the blastocyst, which attaches to the endometrium about six days after fertilization. This is called implantation. By the eighth day, a protective membrane called the *amnion* forms, and as the embryo grows, the amnion entirely surrounds the embryo, making a cavity that will fill with amniotic fluid. This fluid is a shock absorber for the fetus, preventing adhesions when the fetus's skin rubs or bumps against the tissues around it. The fluid also regulates fetal body temperature. (The amnion generally ruptures right before birth—women often refer to it as "my water breaking"—and the fluid is expelled from the mother.)

Day 14

This pivotal day is when, on average, the embryo develops enough to produce hormones that protect it by suppressing the mother's menstrual cycle. That prevents her from having a period, and the remaining fertile ground (uterine lining) provides the environment needed for the embryo's development.

Day 18

Around this time the eyes begin to develop. The baby's heart is also starting to develop.

Day 18 to Day 28

Your baby's heart begins to beat around day twenty-four. The brain, spinal cord, and nervous system are developing now, too. At the beginning of the third week the central nervous system appears.

Day 30

This is an important anniversary for the embryo, as he or she has grown about 10,000 times since conception and measures about 0.6 centimeter, or $3/16$ of an inch, in length. The ears, nose, and eyes aren't visible yet, but the backbone and vertebral canal form by the end of the first month. The tiny buds that will become arms and legs form. The heart is pumping and blood is flowing in blood vessels.

Day 35 to Day 40

The master gland in the brain, called the pituitary gland (which controls the thyroid, adrenal, and male or female hormones for a lifetime), develops now. Other parts of the head are developing, including the ears, nose, and mouth. At this point the heart has an energy output equivalent to 20 percent of an adult heart.

Day 42 to Day 45 (Week 6)

The precursors of teeth are forming. The brain is now functioning and begins to coordinate muscle movements. Brain waves can be recorded. Reflexes are also starting, and if your baby is a boy, the penis is beginning to form. Your baby is moving spontaneously on its own, though it is still small enough for its movements not to be noticed; some moms, however, report sensing its presence. This is the time when mothers miss their second period.

Week 7 to Week 8

Your baby is becoming well proportioned during this time. By the end of week 8, its length is $1\frac{1}{4}$ inches, yet it weighs a fragile $\frac{1}{30}$ of an ounce. The heart is beating steadily, and red blood cells are being produced. The stomach is creating digestive fluids, and kidneys are starting to work. Arms and legs become distinct, and fingers and toes are well formed. Bone formation begins. More and more processes are being performed by your baby. It is even developing taste buds, its tender little lips are sensitive to touch, and its ears are taking on the shape of mom's, dad's, or grandparents' ears.

Week 9 to Week 11

The baby begins to suck its thumb, and its little fingernails begin to grow. The body is sensitive to touch, and he or she can frown, swallow, and even squint. Believe it or not, by week eleven your baby can even smile as it nestles in your womb listening to the soothing sound of your heartbeat.

Week 12 to Week 13

This is a very active phase. Your baby is now capable of kicking, curling fingers and toes, making a fist, turning its head, and opening and closing its mouth. As it prepares for the big world outside, it begins practicing breathing. By the thirteenth week, your baby has fully formed vocal chords, but can't cry because there's no air to pass by the chords. The heartbeat can be detected by the end of the third month, and urine begins to form at the same time. The baby is about 3 inches long and weighs about 1 ounce by the end of month three.

Placenta development is completed by the third month. Shaped like a flat cake when fully developed and formed from parts of the embryo and the endometrium, the placenta allows nutrients and oxygen to diffuse into fetal blood from the mother's blood. Waste and carbon dioxide move from fetal blood to maternal blood via the placenta. Most drugs—alcohol included—pass freely through the placenta. The placenta is a protective barrier against most microorganisms, though some viruses (those that cause AIDS, chickenpox, German measles, and some others) can pass through. In addition, the placenta produces hormones to maintain pregnancy and stores nutrients the fetus will need throughout its development. By the end of the third month, the uterus takes up most of the pelvic cavity.

Month 4 to Month 5

Mom can usually feel the baby's movements at this point. This is also when the baby begins to develop a sleeping pattern, but—just like mom or dad—he or she will be startled awake by loud noises. At the end of the fourth month, the head is disproportionately large compared with the rest of the body, the face takes on human features, and hair appears on the head. Many bones are formed, and joints start to form by the end of the fourth month. Many body systems are developing at a rapid pace. By the end of the fifth month, the head is more proportionate to the rest of the body, and fine hair covers the body. Brown fat forms and produces heat. By the end of the fifth month, the baby is about 10 to 12 inches long and weighs half a pound to a pound.

Month 6

Your baby weighs about $1^1/_4$ to $1^1/_2$ pounds and is about 11 to 14 inches long by the end of month 6. By the end of the sixth month, the baby will begin to gain substantial weight. The eyelids separate and eyelashes form.

Month 7

The eyelids open and close now, and the eyes are moving around, but there isn't much to see. The baby can both hear and recognize mom's voice. Fetuses born at this stage of development (premature babies) can survive, though they still have a lot more fetal growing and development to do. By the end of the month, your unborn baby assumes an upside-down position in the womb. The baby measures 13 to 17 inches and weighs $2^1/_2$ to 3 pounds.

Month 8

Development continues as your baby grows. By the end of the month the skin becomes less wrinkled, and the bones of the head are soft. Subcutaneous (under the skin) fat is deposited, and the testes descend into the scrotum. The odds of survival if birth were to occur at the end of the eighth month are much greater. By the end of month 8, your baby is $16^{1}/_{2}$ to 18 inches and weighs $4^{1}/_{2}$ to 5 pounds.

Month 9

The ninth month has finally arrived. More fat accumulates, and nails extend to fingertips or beyond. The big day—somewhere between 255 and 280 days after conception, usually around day 266—comes, and your little one is born, with mom, dad, family, and friends eager to welcome him or her into the big, new world.

EXPERIENCING THIS JOURNEY

Our hope is that the information in the following chapters, which detail various natural approaches to enhancing fertility—as elsewhere throughout this book—will help you experience the joy of this incredible journey firsthand. Being committed to your health, for the sake of boosting fertility or just because you want to maximize it, takes time, energy, and patience, and trying to sort out the overwhelming amount of information out there can be exasperating. But spend the time and energy, learn as much as you can from this book and other resources, and stay positive. It will pay off, ideally one glorious day when your baby is born.

8

Nutritional Medicine to Enhance Fertility

When you hear the term "nutrition therapy," you might envision a handful of dietary supplement pills. This chapter will review supplements that can help optimize your overall health with a special emphasis on enhancing fertility. However, regardless of what research studies conclude about the benefits of specific supplements relative to fertility enhancement, there is no substitute for a good diet.

We can't overemphasize the importance of what you and your partner put (or don't put) in your bodies. It all stems back to what we learned from Saturday morning educational cartoon commercials (not the ads for sugary, processed cereals): "You are what you eat." So we'll also mention foods to eat and types of foods and contaminants in our food supply to try to avoid. After all, food is your best medicine. Just like a car, your body needs the right fuel in order to perform at its best.

A LITTLE BACKGROUND IN NUTRITION

A healthy gastrointestinal (GI) tract, including your stomach and small and large intestines, is essential to maintaining optimal health. Your GI system is the interface between you and the outside world. The lining of your mouth, throat, stomach, and small and large intestines serve as the very selective and specific filters that prevent large chunks of food from entering into your well-ordered, microscopic internal cellular system. When something adversely affects your ability to absorb essential nutrients or your body's inherent ability to filter what you consume, dramatic and adverse signs and symptoms of health conditions will arise. Things like antibiotics, parasites, and various untreated or improperly treated GI conditions can lead to a cascade of imbalances within the body, including challenges to fertility.

Not all food is good for all people. There are well-documented cases of conditions such as celiac disease, for instance, in which people can't tolerate wheat. Similarly, some cases of asthma are triggered by certain foods. A less evident, yet potentially detrimental food reaction called a delayed immunoglobulin (IgG) response can also detract from the body's overall health. Many patients enjoy more vibrant and symptom-free health when their food intolerances are identified and they can avoid the foods that trigger them.

Due to a delayed reaction, many patients don't even identify the link between foods and the way they feel. They just attribute feeling crummy or tired to the aging process. Thousands of people now enjoy a healthier existence by simply identifying foods that, in the buffet of life, don't nurture their bodies. Now a test to determine allergies can be done at home using a simple kit, which can then be sent to a licensed lab, with no doctor orders required, and the results will be delivered to your home. (See "Nutrition Resources" in the Resources section.)

AVOID ENVIRONMENTAL EXPOSURE

Consuming therapeutic levels of food and following appropriately prescribed supplement regimens can help offset environmental factors. Yet there is no better way to be healthy than to avoid exposure. The old adage "an ounce of prevention is worth a pound of cure" definitely rings true. A study conducted in Malaysia and reported in 2000 showed that exposure to workforce-based risks such as chemicals, radiation, strenuous physical activity, and infections affect reproductive health in women. The effects vary from impacting directly on germ cells or the fertilized egg to altering hormonal balance to inhibiting implantation and development of the fertilized egg. Males can be affected as well; for example, there have been reports of overall increased infertility and increased genetically linked miscarriages.[1] (Refer to Chapter 2 to learn more about environmental medicine.)

One doesn't have to have a high-risk job to suffer the fertility-damaging effects of chemicals. Passive exposure abounds—such as from working in buildings where chemicals are used and are passed through the ventilation system, from living nearby or downwind of industrial and manufacturing plants, and from drinking contaminated water. One can also be exposed to fertility-dampening chemicals by consuming foods that are contaminated. Another big risk still affecting many couples is that one or both partners have been exposed to secondhand smoke, which is high in the element cadmium that can decrease sperm counts and alter fertility levels in both males and females.

These kinds of detrimental effects of toxic pollutants in our environment and food supplies have been known for decades. A study conducted in 1978 clearly showed that toxic pollutants could cause adverse reproductive effects in mammals. We are mammals, along with monkeys, dolphins, seals, and even rats. As we endeavor to live faster, the human "rat race" has created a dangerous environment that threatens our ability to flourish. For instance, in 1950, maleic hydrazide (MH) was introduced into farming practice as a major commercial herbicide and also a depressant of plant growth. MH is used to suppress sprouting of vegetables and other stored food crops and to control sucker growth on tobacco plants. It has been shown to decrease fertility in rats, and plants can convert MH to hydrazine, a well-known mutagen (causing genetic mutation) and carcinogen. Unfortunately, the carcinogenic properties seen in mice and rats seem to reasonably indicate a similar risk in humans. MH is representative of thousands of other such "helpful" chemicals routinely used in the environmental game of Russian roulette, with the equivalent of a six-shooter with three bullets in the barrel. Choosing chemical-free, nutritious foods can improve your odds of achieving and maintaining good health and maximum fertility.

The rest of this chapter is divided into several sections: general nutrition and health guidelines, nutrient support for female conditions affecting fertility, nutrient support for male conditions affecting fertility, and general guidelines for choosing a multivitamin and mineral formula for both men and women.

GENERAL NUTRITION AND HEALTH GUIDELINES

This section provides an overview of diet and lifestyle factors that adversely affect nutritional status. Though it's focused on numerous common vices, which are often points of contention, what a couple chooses to incorporate into their overall fertility-enhancing health plan is ultimately up to the couple and their physician.

Eliminate Alcohol

The scientific literature is clear that both male and female infertility can be improved when alcohol is eliminated from the diet. For males, alcohol consumption has been linked to adverse effects on fertility, ranging from oxidative (free-radical) damage to the DNA in sperm to the potential for prolactin levels to rise. Even small quantities of alcohol have a detrimental effect on sperm quality and, ultimately, sperm quantity.

Similarly, advice regarding alcohol consumption for women is worth considering. The strong link between alcohol consumption by a mother and birth defects supports abstinence. And according to some research, if a woman eliminates alcohol from her diet she can help improve her fertility, for even moderate drinking is linked to infertility.[2]

Stop Smoking

We all know people who smoke and drink and, in spite of these habits, manage to get pregnant. But both these habits should be totally avoided if you and your partner wish to enhance overall fertility and decrease stress on the fetus during development and after arrival.

Research has shown that the more women smoke, the greater difficulty they have conceiving.[3] There is also evidence that when mothers who smoke give birth to daughters, the daughters are only half as likely to conceive when it becomes their turn to try to start a family.[4] Previous generations didn't know this fact; now we do. Stopping smoking is important to your overall health and is one of the best gifts you can give yourself and your future children.

Not just the female half of a couple needs to consider giving up smoking. Cigarette smoking has been linked to decreased sperm counts, increased number of abnormally formed and shaped sperm, and decreased sexual performance. There is also evidence from animal studies that nicotine affects functions within the brain (specifically, the hypothalamus-pituitary axis) that in turn adversely affects the release of growth hormone, cortisol, vasopressin, and oxytocin. This results in inhibition of luteinizing hormone (LH) and prolactin, hormones found in both men and women.[5] Male smokers have been found to have higher amounts of the female hormone estradiol and decreased levels of LH, follicle-stimulating hormone (FSH), and prolactin than nonsmokers, thereby affecting the production of sperm formation. The elevation of prolactin is also linked to decreased sperm motility. This all adds up to fewer sperm with inferior swimming skills.[6]

A study was conducted to measure zinc levels in smokers and nonsmokers. Zinc is so important to the male reproductive tract that its highest concentrations are found here. This study found that smokers had slightly lower levels of zinc, but that, even more important, smokers had higher levels of cadmium, with those smoking a pack a day having substantially higher cadmium levels. Cadmium has been shown to have a highly deleterious effect on male fertility.[7]

Cut Out Caffeine

Virtually everyone likes a little caffeine once in a while, and sometimes more often. According to research, a little caffeine can decrease fertility, sometimes meaningfully so. Coffee and caffeine have been linked to Fallopian tube disease and endometriosis. So avoiding caffeine can help enhance fertility in women. Research points to the consumption of more than 2 cups a day as having an adverse effect.[8] Additional studies have shown that as little as 1 to 1½ cups a day can delay conception. One study showed that even 1 cup can decrease fertility by 50 percent, while other reports say it may take 2 to 3 cups.[9,10] (High caffeine intake may increase the risk of miscarriage, as well, according to some studies.)

Food and drink sources of caffeine include green and black tea, coffee, some soft drinks, chocolate, cocoa, and some medicines. Though not all the studies have shown a correlation between caffeine and fertility, the evidence is strong enough that we recommend eliminating caffeine if at all possible. When in doubt, avoid something potentially harmful, especially if it will help protect a pregnancy. It should be noted that tannic acid in both black tea and coffee, regardless of the caffeine, could have an adverse effect on fertility.[11,12]

Adverse Effects of Dieting

It is not advisable to diet stringently prior to trying to get pregnant. The average adult has a myriad of cancer-causing and harmful chemicals stored in fat tissue. The theory is that when you lose body fat, toxins and chemicals stored in the fat get mobilized. Releasing this potential load of toxic waste into your system while trying to maintain healthy genetic material in sperm and eggs doesn't make good sense. Ideally, sufficient time needs to pass prior to conception to allow the clearing out of these substances. Waiting about six months after dieting and prior to trying to conceive is considered good practice. If you get pregnant before six months, so be it, but actively trying prior to that window is ill-advised, though the jury is still out.

Severe dieting has been shown to cause lowered levels of progesterone, slowing down follicular growth, which in turn can inhibit LH surge and prevent ovulation. Moderate dieting can lead to a small corpus luteum and may increase the likelihood of miscarriage. Your body's nutrient status while dieting may not be optimal for peak nourishment of a baby on board.[13] So if you plan on losing weight prior to pregnancy, it is best not to try to get pregnant until four to six months have passed, to allow for normalization of your body.

Beware of Food Contaminants

The hormones and chemicals in the standard diet of people in the civilized world has been linked to an increased risk of infertility for both men and women. Synthetic estrogens and chemicals, for example, are fairly widely used in the poultry, livestock, and dairy industry. Among other harmful effects, these food contaminants can alter the chemical processes involved in producing the male hormone testosterone (which is found in women as well as men).[14] So consider lowering your intake of commercially available foods and seek free-range, organic alternatives or a fresh salad more often.

Male sperm counts are reportedly declining in Westernized countries, and it is becoming apparent that environmental factors such as exposure to pesticides, exogenous estrogens (estrogens produced from sources outside the body), estrogenlike substances, and heavy metals are all potential contributors. Such factors, individually or in combination, are like the straw that broke the camel's back. They might not be the total cause, but in some individual cases they can very likely swing the pendulum sufficiently to cause pronounced changes in sperm motility and ability to function.[15]

Polychlorinated biphenyls (PCBs) have been implicated as a potentially substantial contributor to diminished sperm quantity and quality. In a study conducted in Asia the highest PCB counts were found in fish-eating urban dwellers, followed by fish-eating nonurban dwellers. In a study of fifty-three males, PCBs were found in seminal (reproductive) fluids of infertile men and were absent in fertile males. There was a correlation between PCB presence and deterioration of sperm count.[16] Another study of fish intake demonstrated that there is a high correlation between lowered fertility and mercury levels, as measured in the hair, and organochlorines (common chemicals found in insecticides like DDT). Fish, including canned fish such as tuna, have been shown to have substantially increased mercury levels.[17] If you are a big consumer of fish, you might want to focus on deep cold-water fish because that water is less likely to contain high levels of PCBs.

But not just men need to worry. There is no question that high mercury levels in women can be passed on to an unborn baby. In fact, the federal government now warns that pregnant women and young children should limit their intake of tuna because tuna contains high levels of mercury, which can damage developing nervous systems. One study showed that maternal consumption of fish for three to six years was associated with lowered fertility. The subjects in this particular study were exposed to PCBs and chlorinated pesticides.[18]

NUTRIENT SUPPORT FOR FEMALE CONDITIONS AFFECTING FERTILITY

The following discussion of the female fertility equation is organized according to various health conditions. Though you may not have a particular fertility challenge, it's important to review all the material, no matter how your case has been labeled. The causes of challenges to female fertility are generally more varied than those of male infertility. They range from sex-hormone abnormalities, altered thyroid function, endometriosis, scarring of the Fallopian tubes, and overall nutritional status, as described in Chapter 5. Working closely with your physician is always important, but it's possibly even more important for women, since whatever steps are needed to promote fertility also affect the environment of a developing baby.

Abnormal PAP Results

Abnormal Pap results are more common in women who are deficient in folic acid, a

B vitamin. This deficiency makes them more susceptible to adverse changes to the cervix from viruses or other causes. Though abnormal Paps are not due to folic acid deficiency, lower levels of folic acid can increase the likelihood that the virus commonly implicated in abnormal Paps will become problematic. An abnormal Pap is a potential clue that supplementation is even more necessary, though all women should supplement with folic acid prior to conception. To summarize, folic acid is needed to maintain cervix health and helps decrease the likelihood of abnormal Pap tests.

The role of folic acid in healthy pregnancies is very well documented. Without sufficient folic acid, a developing fetus is at a substantially higher risk of neural tube defects.

Anorexia

Many women who have struggled with anorexia frequently either don't have regular periods or may not be ovulating, but it is important not to get discouraged. There is no such thing as an absolute, and statistics aren't a certainty. We've all heard stories of people who beat the odds; just think of people who win the lottery. If you or a loved one has suffered from anorexia, treating the resultant nutritional deficiencies is essential. Anorexic women who don't aggressively compensate for past nutrient deficits have an increased risk of miscarriage, premature babies, low-birth-weight babies, and cesarean deliveries.[19,20] Thus, supplementation with a good prenatal vitamin for many months prior to conception and throughout pregnancy, combined with plenty of fresh fruits and vegetables and an overall well-balanced diet, are important. And working with your ob-gyn is always important, but it is crucial when working to increase nutritional status. As you know, with pregnancy comes an increase in the physical demands on the female body because it is now sustaining the growth of a baby. During your baby's development an abundant supply of good nutrition is essential for the proper growth of bone, muscle, nervous system, and heart, as well as for complete maturation.

Past Users of Birth Control and Women Under Stress

If you have taken birth control pills, you are at a higher risk of having lower-than-ideal levels of B vitamins, which include B_1, B_2, B_3, B_5, B_6, folic acid, and a few other minor vitamins. It's generally agreed that taking B vitamins together is best, as they often work synergistically. For instance, B_6 is converted in the body to its active form called pyridoxal-5-phosphate, but in order for the conversion to occur one must have sufficient amounts of other B vitamins, such as B_1 and B_2. Supplementation with a good B complex vitamin or, better yet, a good prenatal vitamin with a nice array of B vitamins would be a good start.

A deficiency of B vitamins can also increase the chance of numerous health conditions, such as depression, altered hormone levels, and carpal tunnel syndrome.[21] In today's world there is an increased need for extra B vitamins because they help us cope with stress. This is why they are called "stress vitamins." Acute and chronic stress alters the biochemistry of the body and generally makes both male and female bodies less fertile.[22] Similar effects of stress can be seen in any given species in the animal kingdom: birth rates soar when there are few ecological challenges and decline when stress is endured. Beyond fertility, stress is believed to contribute directly and indirectly to many chronic degenerative illnesses.

Inflammatory Bowel Disease (Ulcerative Colitis/Crohn's Disease)

Inflammatory bowel disease and other gastrointestinal disorders affect the proper absorption of essential nutrients. Working with your physician and a nutritionally oriented physician, as necessary, is a good idea if you suspect or know that you have such a condition. The replenishing of nutrients is critical to enhancing fertility, promoting a healthy pregnancy, and providing sufficient ability to nurse. People with inflammatory bowel disease who are taking medications such as sulfasalazine can have low folic acid levels that should be improved before getting pregnant.

Yeast Infections

Many women suffer from a vaginal yeast infection sometime during their lives. Such an infection results from the overgrowth of yeast any place in the body. It can arise from a number of different circumstances: an excess of sugar, such as with diabetes; intercourse with someone with a yeast infection, such as jock itch; or antibiotic use when the friendly bacteria (flora) in the gastrointestinal tract have been killed off, leaving an opening for an opportunistic yeast infection.

Boric acid is a natural substance commonly used to treat vaginal yeast infections, but it should be avoided if you want to get pregnant, just to be on the safe side; just because it's natural doesn't necessarily make it safe. Boron compounds are used in the production of metals, enamels, and glasses. Recent studies at the National Institutes of Health indicate that boron may contribute to reduced fertility. So if you suffer from yeast infections, using something other than boric acid would be advisable, so as not to potentially decrease fertility levels.[23] Ask your doctor for safe alternatives.

General Factors Related to Improved Fertility for Women

Some vitamins and minerals are essential for improving the odds of fertility in women, especially iron, a good multivitamin with minerals, and vitamins C and E.

IRON

One research report showed that when women have lower iron levels, supplementation can enhance fertility. This makes sense because without sufficient iron levels, a woman's body does not have sufficient building blocks to optimally produce the new blood supply needed for the developing infant. Getting both a ferritin test and red blood cell analysis called a CBC should always be done before supplementing with iron.[24]

MULTIVITAMIN AND MINERAL SUPPLEMENT

Taking a good multivitamin and mineral supplement, in this case a prenatal vitamin, can help improve fertility.[25] So it's reasonable for most women to start taking prenatal vitamins approximately six months before conception (see more on choosing a formula at the end of this chapter).Working with your physician to find the best formula for you is recommended. According to an article in the *Journal of the American Medical Association* (*JAMA*) in 2002, even adults not seeking enhanced fertility should consider taking a multivitamin daily.[26]

VITAMIN C

A study showed that women taking the fertility drug clomiphene combined with 400 milligrams of vitamin C a day enabled seventeen out of forty-two women who had not previously responded to clomiphene alone to have menses and ovulate.[27] Vitamin C is also a great antioxidant, and it benefits overall health and immune function.

VITAMIN E

In testing, when couples challenged with fertility were given 100 to 200 international units (IU) of vitamin E, the couples experienced significant increases in fertility.[28] In fact, it was believed for many years that vitamin E was so essential for fertility that it came to be called "the fertility vitamin." All worthwhile pursuits of life take heart to achieve, which makes vitamin E even more valuable; this amazing fat-soluble nutrient is also cardioprotective.

ZINGIBER

Zingiber, commonly called ginger, is a popular treatment for nausea and vomiting during pregnancy. Though many women experience no problem when using small quantities of this amazing herb to lessen these symptoms, it should also be noted that some women prone to bleeding during pregnancy or miscarriage should avoid this herb or prenatal vitamins and other supplements containing ginger. That's because ginger can increase the likelihood of bleeding from either the uterus or the placenta, since it works as a blood thinner and is known traditionally as an herb that increases menstrual flow. Sometimes it's better to err on the side of caution.

NUTRIENT SUPPORT FOR MALE CONDITIONS AFFECTING FERTILITY

Decreased fertility in men is often associated with decreased quantity or quality of sperm. You need enough sperm of sufficiently high physical endurance and fitness to accomplish the mission of fertilizing an egg. Beyond sperm quality and quantity, you and your physician will want to rule out the presence or absence of varicoceles, ductal obstructions, or an ejaculatory disorder.

High and low thyroid conditions, low testosterone levels, and other hormone imbalances may also affect fertility. Certain drugs, including, but not limited to, glucocorticoids (like prednisone), nitrofurantoin, phenytoin, and sulfasalazine can decrease both sperm motility and production, or both.[29]

Recent research has shown that male sperm counts are indeed declining, and such environmental factors as exogenous estrogens (estrogens made from sources outside of the body), heavy metals, and pesticides affect the development of sperm, as discussed earlier in this chapter. Fortunately, there are numerous ways to support overall health as the body attempts to combat these hostile forces. Many nutrients have been shown to help both sperm motility and sperm count. These include, but are not limited to:

- Arginine (an amino acid)
- Carnitine (an amino acid)
- Coenzyme Q_{10}
- Glutathione
- Selenium
- Vitamin B_{12}
- Vitamin C
- Vitamin E
- Zinc

Keep in mind that when you're trying to enhance fertility, the process of identifying the cause may be a multistage process. It's like trying to get more horsepower out of an engine; it takes fine-tuning and some patience to get things humming. While it's important for your overall health to identify the causes of lowered fertility, counteracting them will help you maximize longevity and overall quality of life.

Let's review the number of sperm a man needs to produce to be fertile. An average normal semen sample typically has a volume of 1.5 to 5 milliliters (ml), with an average of 50 to 100 million sperm per milliliter, with 20 million being the minimum for adequate fertility. The number of abnormal sperm need to be less than 40 percent, with at least 30 percent demonstrating they can swim in a straight line and not chase their tails (remember: sperm look like tadpoles).

Keep in mind that the process of sperm analysis is still being refined. An interesting report in 1992 showed that 52 percent of men with sperm counts below 20 million per millilter were able to impregnate their wives and 40 percent of men with counts below 10 million per milliliter were also able to impregnate their spouses.[30] Over the last decade there have been advances in sperm count analysis. Tests with a slightly higher predictive value of fertility include the postcoital test, which measures the ability of sperm to penetrate cervical mucus, and the hamster-egg penetration test, which determines the ability of sperm to penetrate hamster eggs. The latter test offers a more accurate reflection of true fertility than a traditional sperm analysis, since it measures the ability of the sperm to successfully complete the goal of egg penetration.

Let's take a look at nutritional ways to help turbocharge your efforts for enhanced fertility.

Sperm Quality

The most important nutrients proven to improve sperm quality are essential fatty acids and vitamin C.

ESSENTIAL FATTY ACIDS (EFAs)

Seek out foods that are high in essential fatty acids. EFAs are critical for the proper consistency of cell walls within your body, including sperm structures. They also serve as a source of energy for sperm.

To review briefly what we learned in Chapters 1 and 2, opposite EFAs on the health spectrum are hydrogenated oils, including cottonseed oil, and any oil that has been heated significantly. Fried foods and processed foods are the main culprits. These oils antagonize the benefits of EFAs and actually decrease the flexibility of cell structures. Visualize an old stiff rubber tire that has been weathered for years (a cell that has been fed hydrogenated oils) compared to a nice, new flexible tire (a cell that's been fed EFAs).

VITAMIN C

The level of vitamin C in the male reproductive tract depends largely on diet. When you eat more vitamin C–rich foods, more C will go to protecting and helping your reproductive system. Lower levels of vitamin C can decrease fertility and increase the likelihood that the genetic material in your sperm becomes damaged. In a study of healthy men, vitamin C intake was decreased and there was a related 50 percent drop in seminal fluid levels and an increase of 91 percent of DNA damage within sperm.[31] Increasing your fruit intake is one easy way to get more vitamin C.

Low Sperm Counts

You've probably never thought about supplementing your diet with cottonseed oil, but if you have a low sperm count, you need to be aware of its deleterious effects. The supplements that have been shown to help boost low sperm counts are coenzyme Q_{10}; vitamins B_{12}, C, and E; and zinc.

COTTONSEED OIL

One of the ingredients in processed food you want to avoid is cottonseed oil. It contains a disproportionately high amount of pesticides, as well the chemical gossypol, which can decrease sperm production. In fact, it has such a dramatic effect on fertility in males that cottonseed oil has been investigated as a male contraceptive. But, like the small print always says, don't try this at home; it doesn't offer a sufficient level of consistent effect, and don't forget about those toxic pesticides.[32]

COENZYME Q_{10}

The energy-giving, vitaminlike compound coenzyme Q_{10} (CoQ_{10}) is concentrated in the middle portion of the sperm and helps produce the energy for sperm motility. Beyond this vital function, CoQ_{10} also serves as an antioxidant, preventing the damaging of the lipid (fatty) cellular structure. Supplementation with CoQ_{10} has been shown to increase sperm count and fertilization rates.[33]

VITAMIN B_{12}

Vitamin B_{12} is important for both RNA and DNA synthesis. Low levels are associated with decreased sperm count and motility. Taking acid blockers or eating a vegetarian diet can increase the likelihood of being deficient in B_{12}. In one study, twenty-six infertile men were given 1,500 micrograms of vitamin B_{12} a day for a period of four to twenty-four weeks. Eight weeks into the study, sperm concentrations had increased in 38.4 percent of the participants and a total sperm count increase of 53.8 percent was noted. Overall sperm motility increased in 50 percent of the men.[34]

In another study, a daily dose of 1,000 micrograms of B_{12} was given to men with a sperm count of less than 20 million per milliliter. By the end of the study, 27 percent of the men had sperm counts over 100 million per milliliter.[35]

VITAMIN C

In a fascinating study, thirty infertile men were given a dummy pill, 200 milligrams of vitamin C, or 1,000 milligrams of vitamin C, daily. Within one week, those getting the 1,000 milligrams daily had a 140 percent increase in sperm count compared to no change in the placebo (dummy pill) group. Likewise, those getting 200 milligrams daily of vitamin C had a 112 percent increase, and both vitamin C groups had decreased agglutination, or sperm clumping. By the end of the sixty-day study every participant who had taken vitamin C had impregnated their partners compared with none in the non-vitamin C group.[36]

VITAMIN E

Each of our cells contains a fatty or lipid layer. That portion of our cells is prone to oxidative damage. Vitamin E helps protect against that damage. In a study of nine men with low sperm counts and decreased motility, there was a significant increase in sperm count and motility when they took supplements of vitamin E and selenium for six months.[37]

ZINC

Zinc serves many purposes within the body and nicely illustrates that the reproductive tract and its functioning often reflect your overall health. In the case of zinc, more than 200 biochemical enzyme processes within the body depend upon adequate zinc levels. When it comes to the male reproductive tract, zinc plays many roles, including testosterone production, sperm motility, sperm production, and overall health of the reproductive tissues. Plus, it's an important antioxidant.

In one trial of men who had been infertile for five years or longer with low sperm counts, thirty-seven men were given 24 milligrams of elemental zinc from zinc sulfate for forty-five to fifty days. The results in twenty-two men were amazing; they showed a significant increase in testosterone and sperm count, leading to nine pregnancies.[38]

Another study of fourteen infertile men with low sperm counts had participants taking supplements of 89 milligrams of oral zinc sulfate for four months. The zinc levels in their seminal fluids became elevated, resulting in improved sperm counts and motility. During the study three pregnancies occurred.[39]

Sperm Motility

Arginine, carnitine, selenium, and vitamin E all promote movement of sperm that is necessary for fertilization.

ARGININE

Arginine is an amino acid that serves as a building block (precursor) for the production of putrescine, spermidine, and spermine, chemicals that are thought to be important in supporting proper sperm motility. A study thirty years ago showed that when 178 men took 4 grams (4,000 milligrams) of arginine daily, 74 percent had improved sperm count and motility.[40] A more recent study using a 10 percent liquid solution of arginine showed that sperm motility increased after six months of use.[41]

CARNITINE

The amino acid carnitine is involved in providing energy for sperm. Sufficient quantities are necessary for sperm motility and are thought to be critically involved in sperm development.[42] When 124 infertile men were tested, there was a direct correlation between semen carnitine content and sperm motility.[43] In a separate clinical study of forty-seven men, results showed that thirty-seven of them had increased sperm motility and an increased total number of sperm after taking 3 grams (3,000 milligrams) of carnitine daily for three months.[44]

SELENIUM

In one study, sixty-nine infertile men were given a placebo, the mineral selenium, or selenium with vitamins A, C, and E for three months. At the end of the study both selenium groups showed significant improvements in sperm motility. A total of 11 percent of the men impregnated their partners during the three-month study.[45]

VITAMIN E

In a study conducted in 1991, oral supplementation with vitamin E was shown to increase sperm motility and resulted in a 21 percent increased rate of pregnancy during the study.[46]

Abnormal Sperm Morphology (Shape)

The shape of sperm is critical in the fertilization process. One substance—aflatoxin mold—has been shown to have a particularly bad effect on sperm morphology.

AFLATOXIN

Aflatoxin is a naturally occurring mycotoxin produced by two types of mold: *Aspergillus flavus* and *A. parasiticus*. Common in nature, *Aspergillus flavus* is often found in grains grown under stressful conditions, such as drought. The mold also occurs in soil, accelerating decaying vegetation, hay, and grains already undergoing decay, and it invades all types of organic material under favorable conditions. Thus, eating grains cultivated by commercial sources or under unhealthy growing conditions increases men's risk of exposure to aflatoxin load that could decrease fertility. In one study of 100 adult males, including 50 from an infertility clinic and 50 who tested normal, the infertile men had more aflatoxin in their semen and showed a 50 percent higher level of abnormal sperm than fertile men.[47]

CHOOSING A MULTIVITAMIN AND MINERAL FORMULA: GENERAL GUIDELINES FOR BOTH MEN AND WOMEN

As noted in Chapter 2, the RDA for most vitamins and minerals is very conservative, and many practitioners recommend taking higher levels of these nutrients in a high-potency vitamin and mineral supplement for optimal health. It should be noted that vitamins and minerals are very safe. The only vitamins that might cause toxicity problems at high levels in healthy people are vitamin A (pregnant women, or those hoping to become pregnant, shouldn't take more than 8,000 IU a day due to an increased risk of birth defects) and possibly vitamin D (400 to 800 IU is commonly recommended for bone health and other benefits).

For women, starting to take a prenatal vitamin six months prior to conception is recommended. Research shows that when nutrients like iron, folic acid, and others are low, conception can be more difficult. According to Katherine Zieman, N.D., the best prenatal vitamins need to be taken in divided doses throughout the day, typically three times a day with meals. Usually, she says, four to six vitamins a day are necessary to get adequate absorption. One-a-day formulas typically do not have enough nutrition—all those little vitamins and minerals take up space—or else they are not bioavailable because the pill is compacted so tightly that the various components are not broken down during digestion and are excreted whole.

Many conventional prenatal vitamins contain iron sulfate as opposed to other forms of iron, notes Dr. Zieman. Iron sulfate causes constipation and, therefore, is disagreeable to a lot of women. For people who have digestive problems even with vitamins split up throughout the day, a supplement containing digestive enzymes, such as papain and bromelain, can help improve absorption.

Some prenatal vitamins contain small amounts of herbs that are thought to benefit women trying to conceive or who are pregnant. Dr. Zieman says that herbal ingredients in prenatal vitamins should be safe, as they support pregnancy, and no reputable company selling prenatal products would risk any possible link to poor pregnancy outcome. "I would not avoid prenatal vitamins with herbs," she says. "My only questions would be if there is enough of the herb to actually be helpful, or is there only enough to make the vitamins expensive?"

Herbs that should be avoided in pregnancy (and keep in mind that you could be pregnant and not know it) are most herbs associated with hormones, such as licorice and others known to cause uterine activity that could lead to cramping and miscarriage, notes Dr. Zieman. One herb that Dr. Zieman likes to prescribe for preventing miscarriage is *Dioscorea* (wild yam) for women who find it hard to carry pregnancy due to low progesterone (though this herb doesn't actually contain progesterone). Another is *Viburnum* (cramp bark) to keep the uterus from cramping during early pregnancy and for hormonal balancing. Herbs that help promote fertility include the herbs mentioned here for hormone balancing, including *Vitex* (chasteberry), which stimulates ovulation indirectly via the pituitary gland, notes Dr. Zieman. You can read more about herbs in the following chapter on botanical medicine. We very strongly encourage you to work with a skilled practitioner with a background in herbal medicine if you have an interest in trying these. If you are undergoing conventional treatment for infertility, be sure to tell your doctor right away about any herbal or nutritional supplements you are taking to make sure they are safe and not likely to interfere with your treatment.

When choosing a vitamin—prenatal or otherwise—it's important to look for natural vitamin E as opposed to the synthetic form. Natural vitamin E is absorbed about twice as well as the synthetic form. Look for "d-alpha tocopherol" on the label; that's the most common natural form of vitamin E. Steer clear of "dl-alpha-tocopherol," which is the synthetic form of the most common type of vitamin E. Here's an easy way to remember the difference: Think of the "d" as signifying that it's delicious for your body, while your body doesn't like the synthetic, or "dl," variety as much. If the label doesn't specify which form it contains, assume it is the inferior, synthetic form and keep shopping.

You also need to know that there are eight different forms of natural vitamin E (four tocopherols and four tocotrienols), and some experts recommend choosing a vitamin that contains "mixed tocopherols" and "mixed tocotrienols" as opposed to only alpha-tocopherol, as the other forms offer health benefits of their own. A supplement containing all eight forms of vitamin E will most likely be the blend clos-

A Success Story

Contributed by Catherine Downey, N.D.

One woman went through the entire fertility gamut and then got divorced. She came to me because she felt her cycles were out of balance from all the hormones she had taken, her periods were irregular and difficult, and she wanted to feel better. I gave her an herbal and vitamin protocol designed to heal the reproductive tract and create a regular cycle, and I warned her that it was also a fertility protocol and she should be careful. She laughed. About a year and a half later she came by my office while on vacation. She had an infant son with her. She smiled, saying, "Remember when you told me to be careful and I laughed? Well, look what happened!"

est to nature. Fortunately, alpha-tocopherol is the only one available in both natural and synthetic forms, so less detective work is involved when it comes to other ones.

Also seek out natural beta-carotene, a vitaminlike antioxidant in the carotenoid family, which the body converts to vitamin A as needed—as opposed to the synthetic form. This form comes from *Dunaliella salina* algae, which should be noted on the label.

Many vitamins are synthetic duplicates of their natural forms in all respects, but it's worth seeking out the natural forms of both vitamin E and beta-carotene, as research has shown they are superior to their synthetic counterparts. Some naturopathic practitioners have an overall preference for vitamins based on whole-food sources, believing they are better metabolized by the body. When it comes to calcium, iron, zinc, magnesium, chromium, and potassium, look for mineral chelates, which are better utilized in the body. Chelates are denoted by words like malate, citrate, carbonate, and other words ending in "-ate," such as aspartate, glycinate, and gluconate.

Focus on the nutrients in vitamins and avoid herbal medicines that some varieties contain unless your skilled practitioner recommends them for specific reasons and in case you become pregnant while taking them.

What's the Right Form and Quantity to Take

Vitamins and minerals come in tablets, chewables, sublingual tablets (which dissolve under the tongue and are absorbed there), capsules, and liquids. In addition to the ingredients they contain, cost, ease of swallowing, and personal preference will help you decide what kind is right for you. Tablets tend to be less expensive, but they can be harder to break down in the digestive tract. Again, a digestive aid may help, or switch to a capsule if this is a problem. Look for vegetarian capsules or tablets if you choose to avoid gelatin capsules.

Nonnutritive ingredients known as excipients are added to supplements to improve consistency or offer other benefits in formulation. The FDA has approved all excipients as safe, but some people may have sensitivities to certain ones (lactose, for example). If you do, look for products free of excipients that affect you. Capsules usually contain fewer excipients than tablets.

Generally, it's best to take a multivitamin and mineral supplement with meals. B vitamins may keep you awake at night, so try to take vitamins early in the day. If you are taking a few vitamins throughout the day, try to start your regimen early in the morning so you don't end up taking vitamins right before bedtime. Always follow the directions on the label. Most of all, remember that supplements are not a replacement for a healthy diet and lifestyle; rather, they are a supplement to your quest for optimal health.

Here are some general guidelines in regard to amounts and forms of nutrients that healthy adults might look for in a high-potency vitamin and mineral supplement. Check with your health practitioner to make sure you get the best product for your needs.

What to Look for in a High-Potency Vitamin and Mineral Supplement

Vitamin A: 5,000 IU and/or 15,000 IU of mixed carotenoids

Vitamin B_1 (thiamine): 25 mg

Vitamin B_2 (riboflavin): 25 mg

Vitamin B_3 (niacinamide): 50 mg

Vitamin B_6 (pyridoxine): 50 mg

Vitamin B_{12}: 1,000 mcg

Folic acid: 800 mcg

Biotin: 300 mcg

Pantothenic acid: 25–100 mg

Choline: 250 mg

Inositol: 250 mg

Vitamin C: 1,000 mg

Vitamin D: 400 IU

Vitamin E (as d-alpha-tocopherol or mixed tocopherols and mixed tocotrienols): 400 IU

Vitamin K: 100 mcg

Calcium (citrate, malate, or carbonate): 1,000 mg

Magnesium: 400 mg

Potassium: 99 mg

Selenium: 200 mcg

Chromium (picolinate or polynicotinate): 200–400 mcg

Zinc (citrate or gluconate): 15–25 mg

Copper: 1–2 mg

Iron: 9–18 mg and up for menstruating women

(Men should opt for an iron-free supplement unless tests indicate anemia.)

Iodine: 150 mcg

Manganese: 2–5 mg

Eating well and taking the right supplements, in addition to having an otherwise healthy lifestyle, may help you and your partner boost your fertility. Besides, these are good habits for a lifetime—they will likely increase your odds of living a long and healthful life, enabling you to enjoy watching your family grow through the years.

9

Botanical Medicine
to Enhance Fertility

You owe your very existence to herbal medicine and plants. Herbal medicine was your ancestors' only medicine. There were no antibiotics except natural, plant-derived ones, and there was no hormone replacement for menopause, just herbs like black cohosh. If it were not for plants, none of us would exist. Plants are the food for the animals we eat, and if you have ever watched a cat or dog go into your backyard or into a field and gnaw on the oddest plants, you'll see that they are usually seeking something they need. Plants serve many purposes, possessing specific nutrients, vitamins, minerals, and also active chemicals that have pharmacological properties within the body.

Some 25 to 33 percent of all conventional medicines are derived from natural sources, including a large number of herbs. Botanical medicine as practiced today also has a multitude of therapeutic benefits that haven't been discovered yet. Some botanical medicines have been thoroughly investigated and active constituents (chemicals) have been identified and concentrated to create "quasi-drug" effects. Others have become pure pharmaceuticals. Yohimbe used for erectile dysfunction has been purified to the active alkaloid yohimbine. The yew tree is the potent source of Taxol, used as a chemotherapy drug, and a species of periwinkle is the source for another chemotherapy drug called vincristine. Foxglove is the original source for heart medicines like digitalis (Lanoxin) and digoxin. White willow gave rise to Bayer aspirin in the 1890s. The list goes on and on.

History speaks volumes about medicinal herbs that often become drugs—potent, lifesaving ones at that. So it's not surprising that they can also be "life giving" when it comes to helping improve conception. Since all medicines have the potential for side effects, working closely with a trained physician to dose and monitor the use of natural medicines is important, especially when dealing with pregnancy.

Technological advances in the herbal industry have brought many difficult-tocultivate plants from around the world to consumers worldwide. Yet, interesting philosophical challenges have accompanied those advances. During the processing of herbal products, when currently identified active ingredients are concentrated to levels above what occur naturally, the therapeutic qualities of the herbs change. A classic example is the fairly recent scare about kava kava in which extracts were linked to a few cases of severe liver disease. However, the vast majority of cases included active constituents concentrated well beyond naturally occurring levels. Thus the question becomes: Did kava kava, the naturally occurring herb, cause the problem or did the use of a quasi-drug extract from a plant cause the problem?

Similarly, there was a report of foxglove toxicity when a person who took the drug digitalis, derived from foxglove, became ill. The point is that a single chemical extract of a plant is not the plant; it is a chemical isolated from the plant. It is traditionally best to use high-quality organically grown or environmentally friendly, wild-harvested (picked from nature) herbs, whenever possible. Using them in their dried or freeze-dried state is the closest one can get to traditional use, unless you are able to harvest the plants fresh and consume them as food, like many of our ancestors were known to do.

Another question that should be considered when processing herbs and performing various extraction processes is whether human knowledge and understanding are sufficiently advanced to clearly identify the most active ingredient(s). Tens of thousands of bottles of the herb St. John's wort, standardized to 0.3 percent hypericin, were sold in the 1990s to people seeking to alleviate mild-to-moderate depression naturally. Later, however, researchers determined that another active ingredient in the extract, hyperforin, was important. If that was not enough to confuse consumers, now there is debate over whether the herb's activity may actually be credited to another portion of the plant. Yet, when the plant is harvested correctly and freeze-dried in a timely fashion, the entire portion of the harvest plant is still present with all the constituents mentioned above, along with all the other naturally occurring chemicals and nutrients, all within therapeutic ranges. The idea that you can't beat Mother Nature or God's creative force is reinforced with such examples.

Herbal products can be purchased routinely in stores as dried herbs in tea form, dried herbs in capsules or tablets, or as alcohol or glycerine liquid extracts. Capsule and tablet forms are available as whole-plant products or as standardized extracts focusing on active ingredients. Your physician or healthcare provider can help you make the right choice for your specific needs.

Often in the practice of Chinese herbal medicine, as with Western herbal medicine, individualized, patient-oriented formulas are designed to treat the same diagnosis. This seems foreign from the Western medical model of naming the disease and giving one drug or, at most, a few drugs to treat the condition. Conversely, there may be hundreds, if not thousands, of combinations of herbals to treat the same basic condition based on the individual patient's specific needs, presentations, and other factors.

APPROACHES FOR WOMEN

There are many approaches to enhancing fertility for women having difficulty getting pregnant. Finding the correct, safe formula for your specific case is important. Also, since what you put into your body can dictate how well a pregnancy proceeds, working closely with a skilled physician familiar with natural medicine is important. Ultimately, what you consume may affect your baby as well.

Altered Cycle or Lack of a Cycle

The individualized approach is nicely illustrated by a study that offered treatment of fifty-three cases of luteal phase (second part of cycle) defect by replenishing the kidney, that is, "the Chinese version of kidney." (Chinese medicine will be discussed in greater detail in the next chapter.) In this study, the fifty-three patients, all with luteal phase defect, were treated with different Chinese medicinal herbs at different phases of the menstrual cycle. On the fifth day of the cycle the treatment was offered with the concept of "nourishing the kidney yin," while invigorating the spleen and replenishing the Qi (the vital energy necessary for life that all people have; pronounced "chee"), supporting circulation, and enriching the blood with the intent of augmenting egg development. Meaningful changes in hormone profiles were noted, and most important 41.5 percent of the women conceived. Sixty-eight percent of these patients, however, required ongoing care to maintain the pregnancy.[1]

CHASTEBERRY *(VITEX AGNUS-CASTUS)*

In a double-blind study of chasteberry, or *Vitex agnus-castus,* fifty-two women with luteal phase defects due to hyperprolactinemia (elevated blood levels of prolactin, a protein made in the pituitary gland that primarily enhances breast development during pregnancy and stimulates lactation) were divided into two groups. One group received 20 milligrams of a *Vitex* product (Strotan) or placebo. During the three-month trial, prolactin release was lowered and luteal phase progesterone synthesis was eliminated. Two of the women receiving *Vitex* became pregnant during the study.[2]

Another study was conducted of 120 women that suffered from polymenorrhea (frequent and often heavy periods), oligomenorrhea (infrequent and scant periods), and corpus luteum insufficiency (disturbances caused by insufficient luteal phase changes in the uterus lining, or endometrium), with 60 percent of the women having previously sought treatment to conceive. They were treated with a *Vitex* extract (Strotan) for six months. Serum levels of progesterone rose from 6.4 to 9.3 nanograms per milliliter (ng/ml). The cycles of a total of 63 percent of the women became normal and 29 percent became pregnant.[3]

HACHIMIJIOGAN

In a study of Hachimijiogan, twenty-seven infertile women with elevated prolactin levels were treated with 5.0 to 10.0 grams per day of the Chinese herbal remedy. Positive changes were seen in fifteen patients who experienced drops of serum prolactin levels. Four of six women that had been experiencing amenorrhea ovulated. Eleven of the participants conceived and delivered, suggesting that Hachimijiogan can be effective in treating women with elevated prolactin levels.[4]

MASTODYNON

Mastodynon, a trademarked herbal combination produced by Bionorica, contains *Vitex agnus-castus* (chasteberry), *Caulophyllum thalictroides* (blue cohosh) , *Cyclamen*, Ignatia, iris, and *Lilium tigrinum* (tiger lily). (Note: the safety of blue cohosh has recently been called into question; it should be used only when prescribed by a trained botanical expert.)

In a double-blind study, thirty-eight women with amenorrhea (painful periods), thirty-one women with luteal insufficiency, and twenty-seven women with infertility of unknown origin were given 30 drops of Mastodynon or placebo two times a day for three months. Fifteen women became pregnant during the three months of the study. What's noteworthy is that pregnancy occurred in the Mastodynon group two times as often as in the placebo group.[5]

Antisperm Antibodies

Sometimes a woman's body treats sperm as if they are foreign invaders and creates antibodies that attempt to kill the sperm. The Chinese formula known as Zhibai Dihuang has been shown to counteract that problem.

ZHIBAI DIHUANG PILLS

This Chinese formula shows promise in helping couples with antisperm or anti–zona pellucida antibodies. In about 81 percent of infertile couples studied, antibodies were converted to negative. Eight couples became pregnant between one and nine months after the antibodies were converted, and antibody negative status was sustained throughout pregnancy.[6]

Elevated Androgens (Testosterone)

If a woman's hormones are not in the appropriate balance and tests show that she has elevated levels of androgens, or specifically testosterone, she may need to take Shakuyaku-kanzo-to.

SHAKUYAKU-KANZO-TO

The herbal combination Shakuyaku-kanzo-to, consisting of an extract of *Paeonae radix* and *Glycyrrhizae radix,* was given in one study at a daily dosing level of 5 to 10 grams for two to eight weeks. In the eight women with elevated androgens (testosterone), serum testosterone levels that ranged from 50 to 160 nanograms per deciliter (ng/dl) were lowered in seven patients to 50 ng/dl or lower. Of these seven patients, six women ovulated regularly, and two of these six patients conceived.[7]

Ovulation Fine-Tuning

Being able to count on regular monthly ovulation is really important when you're trying to get pregnant. You might consider taking the herb *Tribulus terrestris* to ensure that.

TRIBULUS TERRESTRIS

The use of a concentrated form of *Tribulus terrestris* called Tribestan that possesses thirty to forty times the quantity at a level of 45 percent steroidal saponins dosed at 250 to 500 milligrams three times a day for three months, has been shown to help a significant number of women stimulate ovulation.[8]

Adjusting Fertility

Though chasteberry was once thought to decrease the chances of pregnancy, scientific studies show that it, in fact, has the opposite effect. Should you wish to decrease your chances of fertility—lucky you!—increasing the amount of caffeine you drink may steer you in that direction. (But don't count on it, and don't go overboard on caffeine; too much can be taxing to the adrenal glands.)

CAFFEINE

An analysis of 423 couples between twenty and thirty-five years old demonstrated that caffeine from coffee, black tea, cola, and chocolate decreased both the men and women's ability to establish a pregnancy. The higher the caffeine intake among male and female subjects, the lower the odds of achieving pregnancy (that is, subjects with higher caffeine intake had worse odds than those with low intake.[9]

CHASTEBERRY (*VITEX AGNUS-CASTUS*)

According to oral history, chasteberry was used by monks to remain chaste. Strangely enough, it now appears that this herb may actually enhance fertility by inhibiting prolactin levels when these levels are a problem.[10]

Summary of Thoughts Regarding Female Fertility

Traditional use of herbal medicine upholds the concept that one must nurture and nourish the body to achieve wellness. The application of herbal medicine often does not directly treat a specific health issue so much as it supports regaining control of the physiological "functioning" of a body system that may have needed some fine-tuning.

Thus, the herbals recommended for women in this chapter can be used to nurture and nourish the body, allowing it to perform at its peak, yielding a "health solution" via the foundation of true wellness. Treated naturally, many health conditions experienced by both females and males that are not fully explored within this book can be improved and can contribute to enhanced fertility.

CONSIDERATIONS FOR MEN

What affects the man when it comes to fertility is as important as what affects the woman. Fortunately, many herbal remedies are readily available. Working with a skilled physician well versed in natural medicine will help you find the correct, safe formula to solve your specific problem.

Erectile Performance

Several herbals and nutritional supplements can improve erectile performance. Clinically, the way to look at the male reproductive system (as well as the female reproductive system) is as a barometer of overall health. If a person is well nourished, has a healthy nervous system and cardiovascular system, possesses a good mental attitude, and has not been deluged by infection or toxic exposure, the reproductive tract works well in the vast majority of people.

When it comes to male sexual functioning, a man needs sufficient circulation to cause penile engorgement for a firm erection. The best way to accomplish this is to maintain a healthy circulatory system with a great or, at least, reasonably good diet and regular exercise. Yet, the statistics speak for themselves: By the age of fifty some 50 percent of men are having at least an occasional problem when it comes to performance. Poor circulation to the penis can be a barometer of overall cardiovascular health. Taking care of your heart by eating a diet low in "bad" fats and high in fiber is the first step to getting *big* results.

A Success Story
Contributed by Katherine Zieman, N.D.

A patient of mine in her mid-twenties had been told that she would most likely not conceive due to polycystic ovary syndrome. She did not have regular menses and rarely ovulated. I prescribed a combination of herbal medicines and other supplements to balance hormones and support the hypothalamus-pituitary-ovarian pathway. She was also treated with a homeopathic constitutional remedy. She ultimately conceived two children and carried them to term.

GINKGO

Researchers have shown that ginkgo has the ability to expand the blood vessels, increasing blood flow. All things being equal, more blood means a stronger erection. Another benefit of ginkgo is that it can help with memory (you might be more likely to remember having better sex!). Researchers have also found that individuals taking antidepressants, particularly selective serotonin reuptake inhibitors (SSRIs), can diminish the side effects of lowered libido and sexual functioning by taking ginkgo. Consulting your physician prior to mixing natural medicines and drug therapy is absolutely imperative.

MUIRA PUAMA

The common name of this plant-based erectile aid—Brazilian potency wood—says it all. Also known as *Ptychopetalum olacoides*, muira puama, a shrub native to Brazil, has been traditionally used by tribes of that region. According to research in France, it appears to improve both erectile function and psychological excitement.[11] Of the 262 patients complaining of lack of sexual desire and erectile dysfunction who took one to one-and-a-half grams of the extract, 51 percent reported an increase in desire and firmer erections.

BRAND-NAME BLENDS

Trademarked blends on the market include a product called Vinarol, offered by BioNate, and a product called Herbal V, produced by Lane Labs. Herbal V contains vitamins, minerals, and herbal extracts, including vitamins C and E, zinc, selenium, yohimbe extract, yohimbine, damiana, saw palmetto, *Panax ginseng,* and royal jelly.

Patients have reported good short-term results with both remedies. As always, finding the right product for you is important, and consulting your physician is the first step. For more about these and other ways to use natural remedies to heighten sexual functioning for both men and women, see *Better Sex Naturally* by Chris D. Meletis (HarperCollins, 1999), which makes for informative and fun bedtime reading for couples.

Hormonal Improvement for Fertility

Taking an extract of *Panax ginseng* has been shown to promote the development of hormones that aid in fertility.

GINSENG

In a study of sixty-six patients treated with an extract of *Panax ginseng,* those who used the extract had an increased number of sperm per milliliter of ejaculate and improved motility of sperm. There was also an increase in total and free testosterone and other hormones, including 5-DHT, luteinizing hormone (LH), and follicle-stimulating hormone (FSH), and a decrease in prolactin. The research showed that the active chemicals in ginseng, ginsenosides, have various effects on the hypothalamus and pituitary—the master hormone glands in the brain that help control your adrenal glands—the thyroid, testes, and more. This study showed that ginseng directly affected those hormones.[12]

Prostate Fine-Tuning

It is important for all men to remember their prostate gland. Though it doesn't rank in most men's minds as a sex organ, keeping your prostate happy is something you will never regret. It is a ticking time bomb for many men. As men age, the prostate gland begins to swell and enlarge. For too many men, prostate cancer becomes a reality. Problems with the prostate can also hamper peak performance when it comes to sexual intercourse.

All men aged forty and over should get an annual PSA (prostate specific antigen) test. PSA is an indicator of prostate health and a screen for prostate disease. It's also important for men to take nutrients like lycopene, a tomato extract that helps protect the prostate, as well as selenium, zinc, and vitamins C and E. Good sources of lycopene include cooked tomato products eaten with a source of healthy fat, such as olive oil, to enhance absorption. Tomato sauces used on pasta and pizza, for example, can be excellent—and tasty—sources of lycopene.

From an herbal perspective, saw palmetto, either alone or blended with *Pygeum africanum,* is important to help keep domestic peace. That is to say, the swelling of the prostate causes infamous toilet-seat battles. Do you leave it up or put it down? As men age, the flow of urine past the prostate slows, thus the force diminishes and things like nighttime trips to the bathroom, dribbling, forked streams, and the like become a part of life—that is, if you don't do something about a swollen prostate. Flower pollen can help promote prostate health, and the herbs saw palmetto and *Pygeum africanum,* along with zinc, have been shown to help keep in check the conversion of testosterone to 5-DHT, which triggers the growth of the prostate.

FLOWER POLLEN (CERNILTON)

Flower pollen can help you get some flower power on your side. A trademarked process of specific flower pollen, Cernilton, has been shown to promote prostate health. A representative study that demonstrates the power of flower pollen showed that twenty-five men with chronic prostatitis (inflammation of the prostate commonly due to infection) noted subjective improvement of 96 percent and objective improvement of 76 percent. Use of ultrasound imaging showed improvement ranging from 33 to 100 percent.[13]

PYGEUM AFRICANUM

Research has shown that the plant *Pygeum africanum,* which is as its name suggests is native to Africa, can enhance male fertility and improve secretion from the prostate gland. One study showed that an extract of *Pygeum* induced the secretion of additional prostate fluid in men who had previously had insufficient prostate secretions.[14]

Significant from a holistic health and fertility perspective is that *Pygeum* can be used effectively under the guidance of a skilled health provider to help treat prostatitis and benign prostatic hyperplasia (BPH). In a study, eighteen men experiencing these conditions as well as sexual disturbance were given a daily extract of 200 milligrams of *Pygeum.* Upon analysis at the two-month mark, both improvements in urinary parameters and sexual activity were reported.[15]

SAW PALMETTO *(SERENOA REPENS)*

A study published in the *Journal of the American Medical Association* (*JAMA*) showed that saw palmetto, when compared with the drug finasteride, produced similar improvements in urinary tract symptoms and urinary flow but had less adverse side effects. This excellent review showed that, when compared to a leading drug at the time, the herbal approach that worked by helping the body regulate itself was able to accomplish a meaningful benefit, with fewer side effects. Remember that a healthy prostate is a vital part of the male reproductive tract.[16]

Semen Quality

A traditional Chinese formula has been shown to improve the quality of sperm.

BUSHEN SHENGJING PILL

In a study of eighty-seven infertile men treated with the traditional Chinese formula Bushen Shengjing Pill, forty-nine (equivalent to 56 percent) of the eighty-seven participants' spouses became pregnant. Semen quality was improved in 95 percent of men, and hormone levels (FSH, LH, testosterone, and corticosterone) were regulated either up or down toward normal values.[17]

Sperm Membrane Fine-Tuning

Healthy sperm needed to enhance fertility must have healthy membranes. A traditional Chinese formula has been shown to promote that.

SHENJING ZHONGZITANG

A study using Shenjing Zhongsitang demonstrated that it had a positive effect on sperm membrane surface and fertility. After treatment, sperm membranes were normalized and receptor levels improved. This study demonstrated conclusively that this herbal product benefited men with sperm membrane dysfunction.[18]

Sperm Motility

Sperm need maximum agility to move through the woman's reproductive system in order to meet an egg in a Fallopian tube. Two remedies have been shown to help motility.

ASTRAGALUS (ASTRAGALUS MEMBRANACEOUS)

In vitro lab tests have shown that a water extract of astragalus increases the motility of sperm.[19] Astragalus, a very popular Chinese herb, is commonly used to combat viral infections and has been widely used to help patients with viral-induced colds, flu viruses, hepatitis, and HIV.

FERULIC ACID

Ferulic acid, a constituent of many plants, has been shown to quench free radicals and increase the chemical messengers called cAMP and cGMP. It has been shown that reactive oxygen species, a type of free radical, actually damage sperm and adversely affect sperm motility. In a study, ferulic acid was shown to increase motility in both fertile and infertile men. Though the study measured the effect of ferulic acid on sperm outside the body, it holds great promise for systemic applications.[20]

Sperm Quantity

A high sperm count is needed to increase the chances of fertility. Several Chinese tonics have been shown to promote the quantity of sperm.

COMPOSITE WUZI DIHUANG LIQUOR

An initial research study found an 84 percent effectiveness rate when Composite Wuzi Dihuang Liquor was consumed by a group of infertile males.[21] The findings of the study reflected that it was effective for mild-to-moderate oligozoospermia (sperm density lower than 40 million/milliliter) but not severe oligospermia (very low sperm count). Composite Wuzi Dihuang Liquor has also shown some effectiveness in helping those suffering from prostatitis, varicocele, and positive anti-sperm antibodies.

HACHIMIJIOGAN

In one study, fifty-three men with infertility were treated with a dose of 7.5 grams of Tsumura Hachimijiogan for an average of 144 days. Sperm counts rose to above 10 million per milliliter in 41.5 percent of the men. The sperm motility efficiency index (SMEI) was improved in forty (that is, 75.5 percent) of the fifty-three participants. Statistically significant improvements were observed in sperm density, sperm motility, and SMEI. During the study four patients' spouses conceived.[22]

HOCHU-EKKI-TO

Men with low sperm counts when treated with oral Hochu-ekki-to in a study demonstrated improvements in sperm concentrations, rate of motility, and total counts of normal spermatozoa. An overall improvement was seen in 51 percent of the men and 20 percent of the patients' spouses became pregnant.[23]

Varicocele

While varicocele (dilated veins around the testicles) is the most common abnormality found in men and can be surgically and nonsurgically corrected, it can also be treated using Chinese medicine.

TRIBULUS TERRESTRIS

Tribulus terrestris is a plant that grows in many tropical and temperate (warm) areas of the world. The Greeks used it as a diuretic and mood enhancer, and indigenous peoples of South America used it as a diuretic, antiseptic, and anti-inflammatory. The Chinese used it for a variety of liver, kidney, and cardiovascular diseases, and people of Bulgaria used it as a sex enhancer and to treat infertility. Recently, Eastern European athletes have used it to heighten athletic performance. This herb appears to improve sexual function. In one study, a brand-name product containing tribulus called Tribestan was taken by thirty males with varicocele and oligoasthenospermia (low sperm count) for thirty days. The men with varicoceles experienced improved sperm motility, and males with oligoasthenospermia demonstrated increased sperm velocity.[24]

10

Traditional Chinese Medicine: Ancient Wisdom for Fertility

I magine yourself on the Great Wall of China, your feet dangling over the edge—not in the second millennia A.D. but in 200 B.C. For this moment you are in ancient China, and the wall has been recently constructed. The view over the pristine valleys and mountains is indeed a sight to behold. As with many ancient cultures, the people you observe seem at one with the awe-inspiring nature surrounding them. It is from these deep and ancient roots, literally and figuratively, that generations of medical practices based on a oneness with nature were spread. Now they are at our disposal in an often chaotic and unharmonious world. Let's explore the secrets—through traditional Chinese medicine (TCM)—that have given rise to the country with the largest single population in the world, the People's Republic of China. What you learn in this chapter might help improve your fertility—and eventually increase the population of your own family.

BACK TO BASICS

Traditional Chinese medicine is based on 5,000 years of experience and application rooted in Confucian, Taoist, and Buddhist philosophies. TCM views the human body as a whole, interdependent, working system and as part of nature. People are understood in TCM as a microcosm, a "mirror" of the larger universe, or macrocosm. "Looking at the body this way, Chinese medicine uses an entirely different vocabulary rife with symbolism and understandings to explain imbalances in the body," explains Tamara L. Staudt, N.D., M.S.O.M., an acupuncturist with a master's degree in oriental medicine who is in private practice and also runs the Classical Chinese Medicine Teaching Clinic, a clinical training site for the Masters in Oriental Medicine program at the National College of Naturopathic Medicine in Portland, Oregon.

When harmony in the body is disrupted, disease occurs. Several therapies are used to restore harmony: Chinese herbal medicine, acupuncture and moxibustion (a therapy using the burning of moxa, dried mugwort, to produce heat and warm the body to activate its natural energy), Chinese massage and acupressure, mind/body exercise, and Chinese dietary therapy. In acupuncture treatment, thin, sterile needles are inserted into the skin at specific meridian points along the body both to stimulate energy, encouraging balance of hormone function and organ interaction, and to provide pain relief. Acupressure stimulates energy and relieves symptoms with massage and hand-and-finger pressure on meridian points and channels on the skin. Unlike acupuncture, acupressure does not use needles, so it is more limited in the degree and kinds of conditions it can help.

TCM is based on the fundamental concepts of yin-yang and the Five-Element Theory. These two concepts are believed to explain the phenomena of nature and universal changes. According to TCM, the universe is a whole that is balanced with the energies of two opposite components, yin and yang. Yin is usually associated with inactivity, the cold and dark; yang is typically connected to activity, heat, and light. All the body's physiological processes and disease symptoms can be identified on the basis of yin and yang characteristics. In a healthy person, these two components are relatively balanced. When yin or yang is deficient or in excess in the body, a state of imbalance occurs. Having symptoms of menopause, such as night sweats or hot flashes, is an example of a yin deficiency syndrome. Hypothyroidism, in which the thyroid gland is underactive, is a typical yang deficiency syndrome, with symptoms including pale color, edema (swelling), and cold limbs.

The Five-Element Theory, also called the five-phase theory, sees the universe as made up of five elements: wood, fire, earth, metal, and water. These link together relationships between the human body and the environment and among the internal organs. An acupuncturist might needle points corresponding to the five elements to calm or reinforce energy in specific areas, thereby restoring balance.

One of the main components of TCM is Qi (pronounced "chee"), the vital energy necessary for life. Blood, body fluid, Zang-Fu (internal organs), and Jing-Luo are others. Jing-Luo governs the body's meridian and collateral systems, or pathways, whereas Qi and blood circulate through the entire body to maintain balance.

TCM practitioners also use The Eight Principles system to categorize diseases or imbalanced states. The eight are made up of four pairs of polarities, including interior/exterior, hot/cold, deficiency/excess, and yin/yang. Together, they determine disease location, the nature of the imbalance, the presence or absence of a pathological (disease) factor, and the strength of the body's own energies. "Chinese medicine explores and identifies these disharmonies and their source, then uses methods to help reestablish balance," Dr. Staudt explains. "Its focus is returning to whole, not suppression or masking."

Building up Qi, or essence, is not enough to maintain good health, says Dr. Staudt. There must also be balance. It's analogous to conditions in a creek in the sense that problems can develop if there's insufficient water. Yet simply replenishing water may not be enough to restore balance. The water can become backed up and stagnant if a blockage has occurred, creating an odor and becoming a breeding ground for disease.

PHYSIOLOGY IN TCM

It's important to have at least a general knowledge of how TCM views the physiology of the body to understand this system's approach to enhancing fertility. According to TCM, each of us is born with a certain amount of "prenatal energy." This energy, combined with that received postnatally, is what we draw on throughout life. For about the first six years of life the digestive functions are maturing. Digestive function, combined with breath, is critical in the transformation of food and water to usable energy, or postnatal Qi. If we can't receive and transform energy from food, water, and air, we will use up more quickly the finite prenatal stores with which we were born. From about age seven to age fourteen, extra Qi and blood stores begin to build, with proper development and maturation of digestive function. The surplus of these Qi and blood stores becomes the first menstrual flow, called the *tian gui,* or "heavenly water." Tian gui also refers to the monthly menses, which is considered a combination of blood and vital essence in Chinese medicine. When there's no longer a surplus of Qi and blood, menopause occurs.

Three primary viscera, or internal organs, are involved in blood production: the heart, kidney, and spleen. One function of the spleen is to transform food and water essence and send it to the heart. In Chinese medicine, the spleen has a function similar to the stomach and digestive organs of Western physiology, which break down food into usable components that are absorbed and sent through the circulatory system for use in the body. "Western physiology has identified the bone marrow as the cellular production factory for red blood cells, one of the components used in the manufacture of blood," Dr. Staudt explains. "The bone marrow is under the jurisdiction of the kidney network in Chinese medicine, so you see the similarity, as it is the kidney network which provides the 'essence' to the heart." The heart receives transformed food and water essence from the spleen and essence from the kidney, and the heart manufactures the blood from this. Then the blood is distributed throughout the body. The liver network is involved in maintaining the free flow of Qi throughout the body. The Qi moves the blood throughout the body, and the excess Qi and blood is stored in special vessels. One of these vessels is called the *ren mai,* or conception vessel. Ren mai and *chong mai* (penetrating vessel) are the main channels used for storing excess blood and delivering it to the uterus. When these stores are full, excess is delivered to the uterus, and menstruation occurs. In Chinese medicine, menstruation takes place when there is an overflow of abundant Qi and blood in the uterus. The liver opens the gate to allow for menstrual flow, and the kidney is involved in closing the door at the end of menses. Overactivity in the liver meridian can lead to excess opening of the door and release of essence, resulting in miscarriages. Weakness in the kidney's ability to close or hold the essence can also cause miscarriage.

During the first seven days of the menstrual cycle, the uterus empties the blood that has accumulated in the uterus. Free flow of this blood depends on the transport function of Qi, and the liver controls Qi movement. From days seven to fourteen, the body begins rebuilding the stores of blood, which have been depleted. During days fourteen through twenty-one, blood is full and cycled throughout the body, nourishing it. Blood moves to fill the uterus from days twenty-one to twenty-eight. If the Qi is stagnant (not flowing well), PMS symptoms—such as breast fullness, distention of the stomach—can result. If the spleen is weak, it can't transform essence needed to contain blood in vessels and can lead to early or profuse menses. So the first half of the menstrual cycle is focused on blood. After its release, the focus is on rebuilding. The second half of the cycle is more focused on Qi aspects, or the movement of blood throughout the body.

The role of the uterus is to store and discharge—to store menstrual blood and discharge it monthly and to store a fetus and discharge it at term. The blood and Qi are the fundamental components that allow the uterus to function this way. Excesses or deficiencies of either affect the uterus's capacity. According to Chinese medicine, menstruation and conception depend on having sufficient blood from the heart and kidney essence. The uterus is viewed as the junction between the heart and kidney.

CHINESE MEDICINE AND INFERTILITY

Chinese medicine has an impressive track record when it comes to treating functional infertility such as menstrual disorders, endometriosis, and endocrine problems. Structural infertility—an undeveloped uterus, for example—is more difficult. "Infertility will always have some imbalance in the chong/ren meridian," says Dr. Staudt. "This is generally due to some type of alteration in the flow of Qi and/or blood and is often expressed as disorders in the menses." Western medicine often uses hormones to regulate periods, but Chinese medicine offers other alternatives to support the body and reestablish harmony. Treatment usually focuses on the liver, kidney, and spleen meridian networks, since these have direct connections to the chong mai, ren mai, and the uterus.

"In general," says Dr. Staudt, "infertility in younger women is often more of a flow problem, and the focus may be more on the liver network." In women over forty, the focus is more on the kidney because tian gui and kidney essence become depleted with age. One exception is kidney essence depletion at an earlier age due to heavy oral contraceptive use.

According to Chinese medicine, liver Qi constraint or stagnation is one cause of infertility. The liver normally maintains the free flow and movement of Qi through the body. Constraint leads to Qi stagnation, which can lead to blood stasis. The cause of this kind of problem is often unresolved emotions, a high-stress lifestyle, and type A personalities. PMS symptoms—depression, distention, breast tenderness, irritability, and painful menses—as well as blood clots, irregular menses, and irregular amount of blood discharged are common with constraint of liver Qi.

Another type of infertility is caused by kidney essence deficiency that is either acquired or congenital. The two kinds of kidney essence deficiency are Ki Qi and yang deficiency. Kidney essence deficiency can result in blood deficiency in chong and ren and infertility due to cessation of the menses. If menses continue, the essence may be depleted enough that the woman's essence is unable to "grab" the man's essence, meaning that there is no penetration of the egg by the sperm. Excess sexual activity, abortions, miscarriages, oral contraceptive use, and lifestyle can lead to kidney essence deficiency. Dr. Staudt notes that kidney essence deficiency is rarely seen in young women in China but is common in American women. Apparently, part of the difference is related to the use of birth control pills; taking exogenous hormones (hormones made outside the body) tends to deplete the endogenous (inside the body) hormone supply and kidney essence. Symptoms of kidney essence deficiency in women include amennorhea or irregular menses, decreased blood flow, pale, dark, or bright-colored menstrual fluid, and low back pain.

Damp phlegm obstruction can cause infertility, too. People with this problem are often overweight. It's easy to get Qi and blood stagnation with a damp phlegm constitution, and an imbalance of chong and ren can result. Symptoms include very irregular cycles, long intervals between menses, and decreased amount of blood flow or dark blood.

Yet another cause of female infertility is blood stasis. This can result from catching a cold during the first month after giving birth, or intercourse during menstruation, when the reproductive system is open and vulnerable, allowing for the potential invasion of disease-causing factors. Painful menses, blood clots, and dark blood are symptoms of blood stasis.

Male infertility can also be caused by a deficiency of kidney essence, which may manifest itself in such symptoms as fatigue, lack of strength, weak legs, lack of sexual desire, and a pale tongue with a thin white coating. Dr. Staudt also points out that men who ejaculate frequently, either through excessive sexual activity or masturbation, can rapidly deplete their kidney essence, as the ejaculate contains vital essence. A condition called "damp heat in lower burner" is another cause. The liver and kidneys are the organs that make up the lower burner, and damp heat in these areas refers to stagnant energy that blocks organ systems and limits energy flow. Eating too much sugar or too many greasy or deep-fried foods can lead to damp heat in lower burner, and stress can also cause this condition, notes Haosheng Zhang, M.S.O.M., Lac., faculty member at the National College of Naturopathic Medicine in Portland, Oregon. People typically associate fertility problems with lacking something, but an excess of something (stress or unhealthy foods, for example) is commonly the cause of damp heat in lower burner. It may result in a bitter taste in the mouth, a red tongue with a greasy yellow coating, cramps, and swelling in the lower abdomen and perineum. Acupuncture and herbal medicine are used to clear damp heat and restore energy flow and organ function.

One of the biggest issues for men is their Jing level, a measure of vitality. It can become depleted from excess sexual activity or if they don't get proper nourishment from food. Also, avoiding excessively tight clothing and accessories such as watches and especially belts is important because it can impede the flow of Qi. Advances in nanotechnology research have led to the development of clothing impregnated with supermicroscopic ceramic materials that can reflect Qi back to the body, hence conserving it. Like recycling used materials, conserving Qi is much better than creating it. Companies like Vital Age, a new start-up company in Hong Kong, is making products that allow for the passive use of Qi-conserving products. (See Resources for contact information.)

THE CHINESE MEDICINE PRACTITIONER'S APPROACH

Practitioners of Chinese medicine ask clients specific questions on the first visit to determine what's causing the problem. Here are some of the categories you can expect to be covered should you choose to consult this type of doctor. (Numbers 1 and 2 are specific to men and 3 and 4 apply to women only, while 5 and 6 apply to both men and women.)

1. **Erection:** Is the erection firm? Is the skin taut? Are any sensations noteworthy or changed? Is there any change in the amount of arousal needed for an erection?

2. **Quantity and quality of ejaculate:** Color, quantity, smell, consistency, any notable changes.

3. **Menses:** Color, flow, length, amount, spotting, PMS symptoms, history of hormone or birth control use, emotions.

4. **Vaginal discharge:** If there is vaginal discharge, amount, color, odor, and timing.

5. **General:** Body temperature, digestion, food preferences, thirst, sweat, muscular skeleton (including specific questions about back and knee pain), senses (such as ringing in the ears), chest, sleep (nightmares, waking time), emotions, urination, energy, and skin.

6. **Tongue, pulse, and other physical cues:** Practitioners observe the tongue and feel pulses to get more information to help make a diagnosis and to corroborate other clues. Observing the face and body smell, listening to a patient's voice, and examining the abdomen and fingernails are also typical. External influences that affect the body—seasons, weather, and climate—are also considered.

RESTORING BALANCE

Acupuncture is one form of treatment used in Chinese medicine for a variety of health problems, including infertility. The spine is like a hologram for the body, with all the organ systems reflected there. It's similar to the nervous system connections in Western medicine or the basis of chiropractic manipulations (access to the entire body by way of the spine). Several acupuncture points are commonly used in treating imbalances that cause infertility.

Moxa is used to build up essence where there is deficiency. This special herb is carefully processed and burned and held over a specific point, or moxa "cones" can be placed directly on the point. "The heat and the herb carry a tonifying, deeply nourishing effect into the body," says Dr. Staudt.

Dietary and lifestyle recommendations a practitioner makes to treat infertility will likely include specific foods to nourish the kidney or support spleen function. *Qigong* is sometimes recommended to help reestablish balance and harmonic flow. This ancient Chinese self-healing system moves energy throughout the body, stimulating and increasing Qi toward healing. Qigong includes gentle movement, standing and/or sitting postures, and work with breath, visualization, and sound.

RESEARCH

The concepts of Chinese medicine and treatments described here may at times seem esoteric, but a growing body of published scientific research demonstrates the effectiveness of this ancient form of medicine for treating infertility. Here's a look at some of the promising findings.

Acupuncture for Female Infertility

- In a recent study, auricular (at the ear) acupuncture was found to be a valuable alternative to hormone therapy for female infertility due to hormone disorder.[1]

- In another study of twenty-seven women whose infertility was due to hormone disorders, subjects receiving auricular acupuncture had subsequent pregnancies comparable to those achieved by hormone therapy.[2] Researchers noted that acupuncture deserves to be more widely used due to the lack of side effects, low miscarriage rate, and positive effect on patients' general condition.

- In a study investigating the effects of an average of thirty acupuncture treatments on thirty-four patients suffering from ovulatory dysfunction, patients' symptoms improved to varying, but significant, degrees. Acupuncture may adjust hormone levels, bringing them to normal. Based on these results and other studies, researchers concluded that acupuncture may adjust endocrine function, thus stimulating ovulation.[3]

- Results from a recent German study demonstrated that adding acupuncture to the treatment of in vitro fertilization (IVF) patients significantly enhanced their odds of becoming pregnant. Thirty-four out of eighty patients who received acupuncture treatments (one before embryo transfer to the uterus and one after) became pregnant. Of eighty IVF patients not receiving acupuncture treatment, only twenty-one became pregnant.[4]

A Success Story
Contributed by Katherine Zieman, N.D.

A new patient, a woman in her early forties who was planning a pregnancy and wanted to work on her general health, was having regular menses but was not ovulating and was diagnosed with adrenal fatigue. She was placed on a regimen of adrenal support supplements and herbs, she changed her lifestyle to relieve stress, and she had regular acupuncture treatments. She basically reorganized her life to include everything helpful to conception and deleted everything that would reduce her chances of achieving a pregnancy. She started ovulating regularly after about six months of treatment and went on to conceive and carry a child to term.

Acupuncture for Male Infertility

- In a study of men with below-normal fertility, those who received acupuncture experienced significant increases in sperm quality (concentration and motility), with the exception of volume. Researchers found no psychological changes in subjects following treatment, leading them to believe that the positive effect of acupuncture on sperm quality isn't due to a placebo effect, but rather to the acupuncture itself.[5]

- Semen samples of sixteen acupuncture-treated patients with below-normal fertility due to sperm impairment were analyzed before and one month after treatment, which was given twice a week for five weeks, and compared them to semen samples from males with low fertility not receiving treatment. Treated patients experienced increased percentage of viable sperm, total motile sperm per ejaculate, and other improvements.[6]

- Of 297 cases of male sterility treated with acupuncture, pilose antler essence injection and oral doses of Chinese materia medica (Chinese medicines based on indications and dosage detailed in a natural substance encyclopedia), 142 cases (about 48 percent) were cured and 81 cases (about 27 percent) were markedly improved. This combined treatment was also considered effective in another 53 cases (about 18 percent) and ineffective in 21 cases (about 7 percent).[7]

- In a study investigating the effect of acupuncture on twenty patients with very poor sperm density compared to a control group, several patients who received acupuncture experienced improved sperm production. Males with genital tract inflammation showed the most remarkable improvement in sperm density.[8]

Chinese Formulas for Female Infertility

- In an analysis of sixty women experiencing infertility due to defects in the luteal phase of the menstrual cycle, Chinese herbs known to tonify the kidney and regulate menstrual cycles were found to improve cycles following treatment. The pregnancy rate in thirty-two uncomplicated cases of luteal phase defect was 56 percent. Coordinating yin and yang and regulating Qi and blood were among the key points of this treatment.[9]

- In a study of fifty-three patients with luteal phase defect treated with different Chinese medicinal herbs at different phases of the menstrual cycle for three cycles, patients experienced significant luteal phase improvements. The findings suggest that Chinese herbal medicines capable of replenishing the kidney could improve luteal function. Out of fifty-three cases, twenty-two (41.5 percent) conceived, but 68.18 percent of them required other measures to preserve the pregnancy.[10]

- Forty-six patients with endometriosis were treated with TCM by removing blood stasis, resolving phlegm, and softening and resolving lumps. According to TCM, endometriosis is a disease of blood stasis and mass in the lower abdomen. The effectiveness rate was 91.3 percent, and six of ten infertility patients in the group became pregnant.[11]

- In another study, seventy-six endometriosis patients were treated with a TCM prescription called "endometriotic pill number 1," with rhubarb as the main ingredient. The total effectiveness rate was 80.26 percent, with symptom relief ranging from decreased pelvic and intercourse pain to diminished size of mass or nodule and decreased dysmenorrhea (difficult menstruation that is often painful). Three cases, or about 13 percent, of twenty-two infertility patients in the group got pregnant.[12]

- TCM medicines for replenishing kidney, combined with acupuncture, for one to three months induced ovulation in female patients experiencing anovulation (failure to ovulate) in a recent study. Twelve of twenty-three patients with anovulation complicated with infertility became pregnant, leading researchers to conclude that replenishing TCM kidney medications combined with acupuncture treatment could be effective in treating infertility due to anovulation.[13]

- Zhibai Dihuang Pill, a recipe of Chinese medicinal herbs, was used in a study to treat infertile couples with antisperm and/or anti–zona pellucida antibodies in their blood serum. (See Chapters 5 and 6 for more information on these conditions.) After treatment, the antibodies were negated in about 81 percent of the infertile couples. Eight cases of successful pregnancy occurred in one to nine months after antibodies became negative, and the negative status was maintained throughout pregnancy.[14]

Chinese Formulas for Male Infertility

- Among eighty-seven infertile male patients with abnormal semen who were treated with Bushen Shengjing Pill, semen quality was enhanced following treatment, and forty-nine spouses (56.32 percent) of treated patients became pregnant. The medication regulated hormone levels, restoring them to normal values.[15]

- In a study of thirty-seven infertile patients with varicocele (a collection of dilated veins in the scrotum, most occurring on the left side but as many as 20 percent occurring on both sides) who were treated with Guizhi-Fuling-Wan (7.5 grams/day) for at least three months, sperm concentration and motility were improved in the majority of patients. Varicocele disappeared in forty out of fifty patients, a disappearance rate of 80 percent. Researchers concluded that Guizhi-Fuling-Wan is considered effective for improving circulation disorders in varicocele and semen quality.[16]

- A Chinese herbal medicine called Hochu-ekki-to was administered for over twelve weeks to forty-five male patients with infertility due to oligozoospermia (sperm density lower than 40 million/milliliter). Significant increases in sperm concentrations, movement, and total count of normal sperm were observed (with no serious side effects), especially among patients with moderate oligozoospermia. Nine of the patients' spouses (20 percent) got pregnant.[17]

- A Chinese medicine called Hachimijiogan was given to twenty-eight men with oligozoospermia and seven with azoospermia (no living sperm in the ejaculate) for eight to twenty-eight weeks. Sperm number, motility, and fertility measures were remarkably improved in patients with oligozoospermia but not in those with azoospermia.[18]

- The effects of Chinese medicines Tsumura Hachimijiogan and Tsumura Ninjintoh were compared to the drug clomiphene citrate in male patients complaining of sterility due to both or either oligozoospermia or asthenospermia (reduced sperm motility). After men were given Hachimijiogan three times daily for four months, the sperm count improved in 21 percent of patients with oligozoospermia, and sperm motility improved in 50 percent of patients with asthenospermia. After men were given Ninjintoh three times daily for four months, the sperm count improved in 31 percent of patients with oligozoospermia, and sperm motility improved in 45 percent of patients with asthenospermia. Both TCM medications were more effective in improving sperm count and motility than clomiphene citrate, and no side effects or abnormal hormone levels were observed in any of the TCM-treated patients.[19]

- Thirty infertile male patients were given a traditional herbal medicine called Goshanjinkigan (that's its Japanese name, as it is used in that country, too; in Chinese it's *Niu-che-shen-qi-wan*) daily for three months or more. Sixteen patients showed significant improvement in sperm motility, and ten patients experienced an effective increase in sperm count. One patient's spouse became pregnant during the treatment period.[20]

NEED TO RESTORE BALANCE

You will agree that TCM has some impressive research proving its effectiveness in treating various types of infertility in men and women. If you're interested in learning more about this ancient, effective, and safe system of medicine, or if you'd like to seek out a qualified practitioner, refer to the Resources section at the back of this book. Several Chinese herbal formulas (Bushen Shengjing Pill, Composite Wuzi Dihuang Liquor, Hachimijiogan, Hochu-ekki-to, Shakuyaku-kanzo-to, and Zhibai Dihuang Pills) were covered in Chapter 9, as well, so consider reviewing that section. You may find that TCM offers just what you need to restore balance in your body and to help you and your partner conceive.

11

When Less Is More: Homeopathy for Enhanced Fertility

You've probably heard of homeopathy, but, more important, have you ever asked yourself what makes homeopathy different from vitamin and herbal supplements, traditional Chinese medicine, and other complementary therapies? Often, homeopathy is lumped together with such therapies under one big umbrella, but it is fundamentally very different. Like other forms of natural medicine, however, homeopathy may help boost fertility in some cases. In this chapter, you'll learn about the philosophy behind this safe and effective natural therapy and, more specifically, how you can benefit from it.

THE BIG PICTURE

In homeopathy, remedies made primarily from extremely diluted vegetable, mineral, and biological sources (which are shaken vigorously upon each dilution) are given to promote the body's self-healing to overcome a specific health problem. Rather than acting only on the apparent symptoms of the disease, they act directly on the person. These remedies stimulate the body itself to fight whatever is causing the problem, balancing and harmonizing the whole organism. Enhanced functioning of the reproductive system and increased fertility are among the many positive outcomes of the general increase in health following successful homeopathic treatment. But homeopathy encompasses more than tiny vials of remedies.

"It's really important to understand that homeopathy is not just a type of medicine," points out Lucy Vaughters, P.A.C., C.C.H., who is on the faculty of homeopathy at Bastyr University in Seattle, Washington. "It's also the application of certain principles."

One of these is the principle of individualization, or fitting the way symptoms present themselves in a specific person to the appropriate remedy. For example, one person experiencing the flu might have somewhat different symptoms than someone else with the flu. As a result, different remedies might be indicated for each, even though they may have the same sickness.

Another important principle of homeopathy, says Vaughters, is that of holism, or treating the whole person. Before choosing a remedy, homeopathic practitioners take into account the person's physical symptoms, in addition to a patient's emotional state, belief system, and more. A complete picture of a person's symptoms has to be clear in order to determine the best remedy. According to homeopathy, disease doesn't reside in an organ but, rather, in the whole person.

"There's something pervading the whole person," Vaughters explains. "The body is out of balance, and you have to restore that balance in order to cure the earache or stomachache, for example."

Another fundamental principle of homeopathy is giving the remedy that matches a person's symptoms in the minimum dose that will promote healing. This concept that like cures like, also called the concept of similars, is a cornerstone of homeopathy. Though it may seem a strange solution at first, remedies are chosen that normally cause the same symptoms that the ill person is experiencing. That stimulates the body to overcome disease and illness. The cause of the illness is less important in determining homeopathic treatment than the symptoms it causes.

For example, explains Jay Borneman, a member of the board of the National Center for Homeopathy, when you chop onions, your eyes start tearing and your nose will likely begin to run. In acute rhinitis, characterized by running eyes and nose, *Allium sepa*—the red onion—is used to treat these symptoms, though it actually causes those symptoms in healthy people. A principal homeopathic remedy called *Rhus toxicodendron* (its Latin name) comes from poison ivy, which—in healthy people—causes skin irritation followed by joint pain. Homeopathically, *Rhus toxicodendron* is used to alleviate rheumatic and joint pain (such as that of arthritis), which is made better with motion (such as walking). *Coffea cruda*, derived from raw coffee bean, is useful in calming children who are nervous, restless, and who get overexcited. (Does that sound like anyone you know after one too many lattes?) This concept of similars may seem counterintuitive, but understanding the beginnings of this mysterious medicine helps illustrate it more clearly.

WAY BACK WHEN

Samuel Christian Hahnemann developed the system of homeopathy over the course of fifty years, starting in the late 1700s. While translating a medical text in 1790, he questioned the author's assertion that the drug quinine was effective against malaria because of its bitter and astringent properties. Hahnemann knew other drugs were even stronger and more astringent, but they weren't effective in treating malaria.

Hahnemann, conducting an experiment on himself, took quinine twice a day, and he found that the drug caused malarialike symptoms—drowsiness, trembling, and pulse quickening, among others. From this, he suggested that a drug acts therapeutically when it causes symptoms in someone without the disease that are like those experienced by someone who has the disease. Thus, the concept of similars was established.

Hahnemann and his students tested other common drugs on themselves and other healthy people, noting the symptoms produced. He called these tests "provings." Once a remedy was "proven" in many people, Hahnemann tested the drugs by treating sick people with them. He diluted the drugs to avoid toxicity and side effects and found that they actually worked better in the diluted form than in their conventional form.

Homeopathy was effectively and widely used for the next several decades. It eventually fell out of favor in the United States with the advent of technology and materialism less than a hundred years later. But a growing interest in alternative forms of healing in recent years has caused a renewed interest in homeopathy. This type of medicine is still much more commonly used in some European countries, Mexico, and India than it is in the United States, but it is possible to find skilled practitioners and high-quality remedies stateside.

THE SCIENCE BEHIND HOMEOPATHY

Even though it's been more than 200 years since Hahnemann began his experiments, and even though homeopathy is used by millions of people all around the world, much about homeopathy remains a mystery. One theory is that the water and alcohol used in the manufacturing of homeopathic remedies may store energy frequencies and a kind of memory of the substances from which they are prepared. These remedies are usually so diluted that there should be no remaining molecules of the mother (original) substance present. Even if this is the case, how and why such small doses of homeopathic remedies have health benefits is unclear, although there are several theories. However they work, clinical experience and limited research studies have shown that these remedies do act therapeutically when used correctly.

There hasn't been much research on homeopathy compared to conventional drugs, vitamins, and the most popular herbs. That is partly because the remedies are so diluted that it's not really possible to quantify the minute amount of the active substances within them. Also, the usual clinical study assigns one treatment to a group of people (with a control group receiving placebo) and observes the effects. But, as noted earlier, homeopathy is based on individualization. As opposed to treating all flu or arthritis sufferers with the same treatment, for example, homeopathic practitioners match each individual's symptoms with the appropriate remedy. The one that might improve flu or arthritis symptoms in one person may do nothing for another sufferer. The difference between conventional clinical studies and the way homeopathy is used confounds typical research results, making it a challenge to design studies that offer meaningful results.

There is also a fair amount of skepticism about the effectiveness of homeopathy, so even positive research results are not always enough to convince skeptics. Keep in mind, however, that scientists do not know the mechanisms of some effective prescription drugs, but they are still used because they work well in treating illness. Some people speculate that the placebo effect explains why homeopathic remedies seem effective—that is, because people taking such remedies think they are taking medicine, they will feel better. But the effectiveness of homeopathy in animals and children—who don't know they are taking medicine—seems to negate that argument.

In addition, homeopathic remedies cannot be patented, so there is no incentive for private companies to invest in researching their benefits. That is another big reason that research is lacking. Despite these limitations, research has shed some light on the benefits of this curiously effective, nontoxic, time-tested form of medicine.

WHO CAN BENEFIT?

Homeopathic remedies may be useful in reducing migraine attacks, treating arthritis, ear infections, allergies, asthma, tonsillitis, and other maladies.[1,2] Vaughters considers homeopathy especially useful for patients with chronic (long-term) health problems, many of which cannot be helped with conventional medicine. Among these she counts lupus, PMS, ear infections, migraines, ulcerative colitis, gastrointestinal problems, and irritable bowel syndrome. She stresses, however, that anyone with chronic problems should consult a knowledgeable practitioner instead of trying to self-treat. Homeopathic remedies are commonly used to improve reproductive health and fertility, but the expertise of a skilled practitioner is absolutely essential in choosing and using these effectively. A recent study published in the journal *Homeopathy* demonstrated that the rate of improvement in sperm count among forty-five subfertile men treated with single homeopathic remedies for an average of 10.3 months was comparable to improvement achieved with conventional therapy.[3] Remedies were prescribed based on overall symptomatic situation and sperm density, and the percentage of sperm with progressive and propulsive motility improved significantly, especially among men with oligoasthenospermia (scanty seminal secretion and reduced sperm motility). General health also improved.

For acute (short-term) problems (not fertility problems), such as a cold, a bruise, or the flu, using homeopathic remedies—which are considered over-the-counter drugs, or OTCs, by the FDA—is probably fine, as they are nontoxic. Even so, working with a practitioner is more likely to yield the best results. You can find individual remedies, combination remedies, and kits containing many remedies and directions to help you determine which is best to take. Remedies are available in the form of liquids, tablets, and powders. While a label may only list one symptom a specific remedy is used for, that doesn't mean it doesn't have other applications, as well. Be aware that, initially, homeopathic remedies may make symptoms slightly worse. In extremely sensitive people, this can be a problem, but for most people it is only a slight and passing nuisance, if it happens at all.

In people already taking medications, it's harder to get a clear picture of the true symptoms. That is because drugs can also cause symptoms in addition to those being treated with homeopathy. "For example," says Jay Borneman, "sometimes in older folks you get layer upon layer of drug therapy and corresponding symptoms." This makes it especially important to work with a very experienced practitioner who can determine which symptoms are the result of a health problem and which are caused by other medications. Then, the appropriate remedy can be chosen. Some drugs (like steroids) can interfere with homeopathy, too, so working with a practitioner is recommended to get the best results.

CONSULTING A HOMEOPATHIC PRACTITIONER

As in conventional medical practice, homeopathic practitioners need to know the relevant diagnosis of a patient and the physiological or structural reasons for infertility. The first few minutes of the homeopathic information intake is much the same as the M.D.'s or N.D.'s exploration of tangible symptoms, says Werner Vosloo, who holds a master's of science degree in homeopathy (M. Sc. Hom.). Carefully gather-

A Success Story
Contributed by Katherine Zieman, N.D.

A young woman, aged twenty-four, had her periods stop completely after the sudden, tragic, and violent death of friends in a plane crash. She had no menses at all for over six months. Prior to this, she had never missed a period since menarche. I gave her a homeopathic remedy that specifically targeted for lack of monthly cycles due to grief. Her menses were reestablished within one month with no further treatment.

ing this patient information also helps a homeopath determine whether or not the patient has warning signs of serious disease requiring urgent care or if the problem requires mechanical intervention. The homeopath tries to establish if there is an existing cause of the problem and to ascertain that he or she has done everything possible to find and remove obstacles to a cure. The diagnosis and exact or characteristic way that symptoms manifest themselves are essential to determining the outcome of the homeopathic process and, ultimately, the medicine given to the patient.

But disease is more than a diagnosis of, for example, low sperm count, amenorrhea, or other factors that prevent conception, notes Vosloo. It is an altered dynamic state, outwardly observable via symptoms the body produces. "Painful menstrual cramping, impotence, or abnormal hormonal profiles might be symptoms or causes of infertility, but they are only helpful if given their proper place as part of the larger picture," he explains. Homeopaths look for symptoms of disease in the entire body, mind, and emotional spheres, as well as characteristic symptoms that might not be related to any disease picture but that might help distinguish one patient from another with the same disease. "Hahnemann reminds us to place a lot of focus on the striking, exceptional, unusual, and odd signs and symptoms of disease," says Vosloo. "There are often the weird or quirky things about us that we do not want others to know because they make us different, but those are the most helpful for the holistic homeopath." This complete picture is referred to as the totality of symptoms.

Specific individual symptoms are part of this picture. For a symptom such as a headache, the homeopath needs to know the specific location of the pain (the back of the head and behind the left eye, for example), as well as the specific sensation, like a sharp or shooting neuralgic (nerve) pain. Modalities, or things that either intensify or ameliorate the specific sensations the patient feels, are considered as well. For example, whether or not the sharp headache in the back of the head is lessened when pressure is applied is considered. Symptoms called "concomitants" occur in the same timeframe as the headache or other symptom, but they may not be related to the headache itself. An example could be developing a fear of knives and other sharp objects when the headaches started appearing or when other symptoms are present. Homeopaths also consider the speed of onset or pace of the symptom together with the symptom's intensity. Relative to a simple, mainstream diagnosis of a headache, determining the totality of symptoms is more valuable to the homeopath.

"To complete the picture, we need to have as many different symptoms, constructed as above, as the patient can share with us," says Vosloo. "The totality of symptoms allows you to construct a logical, coherent whole that is the unique expression of the disease in the patient. It must have a central idea or theme that is true to the expression seen in the patient and must be observed and recorded with fidelity. This is more than the sum of the symptoms observed in the patient, because it considers a central theme uniting it into a picture with a characteristic identity. Once you have completed this, you do more than just cover the random symptoms observed in any given case, but you can address the core of the pathology. This is the difference between recognizing symptoms of curative medicines in a patient and observing the pattern or characterizing combination of symptoms found only in the medicine that will be homeopathic to the case."

Homeopaths have to be very good listeners, allowing patients to tell their entire story, uninhibited, so the practitioner can do justice to the interview and observe the characteristic expression of the patient. As the same time, homeopaths must construct a picture with complete symptoms and be on the lookout for individualizing or characterizing symptoms. Some homeopaths prefer very spontaneous consultations, while others prefer structured, guided interviews. The homeopath explores the detailed history of the main complaints, including how they affect the patient's daily functioning.

Vosloo gives the following two fictitious scenarios to illustrate the importance of these details: In one case, Gill and her husband have been trying to get pregnant for eight months and are very excited about starting a family. When Gill realizes that she is starting her normal menstrual flow and is not pregnant, she calls her husband and arranges to meet for dinner at their favorite restaurant. She is very sad and wants to share her deep disappointment with him in a place with people and activity, which always makes her feel better. In the second case, Jenny and her husband have been trying to get pregnant for eight months. She is anxious about starting a family, yet very disappointed that she hasn't been able to get pregnant after trying so hard for several months. When she feels the normal sharp premenstrual cramps signaling she is not pregnant, she is filled with resentment that her husband doesn't make enough money so she can stay at home and not have to work. She phones him immediately at work and tells him how sorry she is that she married him. In both these scenarios, the women are battling infertility, yet they handle the symptoms very differently. Observing the specific way that a person reacts to symptoms is essential in understanding a person and finding a remedy similar, or homeopathic, to the case.

Additional factors that homeopaths consider include the following:

- Other significant illnesses

- Interactions with environment (weather sensitivities, for example)

- Skin (skin tone, eruptions, exzema, temperature, cracks, and so on)

- Quality of sleep, insomnia, dreams, perspiration, teeth grinding, perspiration while sleeping

- Appetite, thirst, food cravings, aversions, and intolerances

- Menstruation and sexuality

- Digestion, stool, and urination

- Fears and phobias

- General energy level

- Mental and emotional symptoms

From this information, the homeopath studies and arranges the factors into a sensible whole, then extracts the most important themes and symptoms and prepares for repertorization (list of symptoms and corresponding medicines). A repertory refers to an index of symptoms found in the *Materia Medica,* followed by a listing of medicines that have the symptom as part of their picture. Modern homeopathic software repertories make this process more efficient, so the right medicine can be found quickly and accurately.

Homeopathy tends to be more effective for problems that are functional in nature rather than structural. For example, homeopathy works well for balancing hormonal or metabolic disturbances and for dealing with problems related to abnormal physiology or biochemistry, says Vosloo. This form of natural medicine works to restore harmony in the body, and it is ideally a long-term commitment. It's not possible to predict how long it will take to cure a given disease, but the general rule is to allow one month for every year the problem has existed. Even so, individual cure rates vary greatly, so that shouldn't be used as a measure to gauge progress. (The Resources section at the back of this book has a list of websites with referrals to homeopaths in your area and other homeopathic resources.)

REALITY CHECK

It's important to remember that, like all forms of medicine, homeopathy is not a panacea or a cure-all. It can be very effective, but it doesn't work for everyone all the time. A person with a chronic condition like lupus may find relief with various treatments (including homeopathy) at various times. But if you have a blood clot blocking blood flow to your heart, homeopathy isn't going to alleviate what surgery will.

Also, if poor lifestyle habits are making you sick, homeopathy isn't going to

How to Use Homeopathic Remedies

Here are some of the most important things you should know when shopping for and using homeopathic remedies:

- Most over-the-counter remedies are 12X, 12C, 30X, or 30C dilutions. These refer to how many times the original substance was diluted. In the decimal (X) system, remedies are repeatedly diluted (and shaken) with one part active substance to 10 parts water/alcohol mix. For example, 6X signifies this has been done six times. C signifies that the remedy has been repeatedly diluted with one part active substance to 100 parts alcohol/water mix; 30C means this has been done thirty times. The higher the number, the more diluted the remedy.

- Look for the letters HPUS on the label. That means the medicine was prepared in accordance with the standards of the Homeopathic Pharmacopeaia of the United States.

- Avoid products that tout outrageous claims or that don't include the Latin names for the contents.

- Store remedies in a cool, dry place (not in the bathroom medicine cabinet).

- Follow label or kit directions for dosages.

- Single remedies are recommended over combination formulas when available and when your choice of remedy is based on clear indications.

- Pour the dose on a tiny piece of white paper or in the bottle cap to avoid contamination.

- Drop the dose under your tongue where it will dissolve.

- Screw on bottle caps tightly to preserve freshness.

reverse the damage you're doing to yourself. And don't go to a homeopath with the expectation that you're going to drop your other medications. Be accountable, be sensible, and be realistic when it comes to homeopathy or any other kind of medicine.

"The great news," says Vosloo, "is that in homeopathy we have a host of remedies that have infertility as a part of the symptomatology, and can therefore guide patients toward a state of general better health if infertility is one of the complaints. Enhanced fertility naturally is inevitably a part of such an outcome."

12

Physical Medicine: Hands-on Fertility Enhancement

The musculoskeletal system is made up of skeletal muscle tissue and connective tissues, and the skeleton serves as the framework that supports and sustains our human form. Healthcare providers who focus on treating the musculoskeletal system practice physical medicine. Some of those trained in physical medicine techniques include the osteopathic physician (D.O.), the chiropractor (D.C.), the naturopathic physician (N.D.), the physical therapist (P.T.), and the occupational therapist (O.T.). There is a saying that offers insight into why physical medicine techniques are important to overall well-being, as well as to fertility: "Structure begets function and function begets structure." Or, put another way, your anatomical body parts serve a purpose, and that purpose determines the optimal space and shape needed to accomplish the function.

You might wonder what conceivable role your bones and muscles have in maintaining or improving fertility. A couple of examples help illustrate the answer. Imagine that you have structural problems with your feet—you are flat-footed, for example. The feet serve as the foundation of your entire body. If your feet don't provide a solid and level starting point, you could suffer from knee pain, hip pain, low pack pain, and even a headache. To take this example a little further, imagine that you have resulting low back pain. Treating your low back directly with heat, massage, and manipulation of the spine might result in temporary relief, but the benefits of such therapies will not be permanent or truly meaningful because they do not address the underlying cause of the problem. In that case, your feet are still out of whack.

Now let's look at low back pain a little more closely, this time assuming that the problem actually begins in your lower back. If you have a back problem that results in the pinching of nerves, such as a slipped disc, this may very well affect more than your level of pain; it could affect how well your internal organs, including your reproductive tract, are working. That's because the nerves that come from the spinal cord that are protected by the bones in your spine connect your brain and the central nervous system to the rest of your body. At each level of your spine (cervical, thoracic, lumbar, and sacral-coccyx), nerves leave through small passageways in the bony structures and connect to various internal organs, including the intestines, ovaries, bladder, and so on. If the nerve supply is insufficient or less than optimal, that may affect the overall functioning of your reproductive tract. Structural changes internally due to scar tissue or other issues may impair the functioning of the affected organs or tissues and, thus, the structure as it was originally intended to function. Providers of physical medicine use hands-on, noninvasive techniques to help you gain enhanced performance from your body, both at the structural and functional levels and as appropriate to your particular case.

Chiropractic is one form of physical medicine that might aid in certain kinds of infertility. Chiropractors identify and, by making manual adjustments, remove subluxations, or spinal misalignments, that interfere with the body's normal functioning. Some forms of trauma that can cause spinal misalignments include occupational hazards, falls and other accidents, poor posture and sleeping habits, and heavy lifting and twisting. Emotional stressors can also contribute.

Subluxations have the potential to affect fertility in several ways. For one, restricted movement of bones in the head or sacrum can affect the circulation of cerebrospinal fluid that is needed to keep the hypothalamus and anterior pituitary gland functioning properly. These glands are responsible for making luteinizing hormone (LH) and follicle-stimulating hormone (FSH), which are both crucial to healthy reproductive function in women. Subluxations can hinder the thyroid gland, leading to hypothyroidism, a condition associated with infertility. Regular function of the Fallopian tubes, cervix, and ovaries might be compromised by subluxations in some cases, too. Men can experience problems related to the functioning of the penis, testicles, and sperm as a result of spinal misalignments. Removing subluxations may help restore proper reproductive function when they are the cause of the problem.

Dr. David Russ, D.C., practices bodywork, including massage, craniosacral therapy, and chiropractic, and serves as department chair of the physical medicine department at the National College of Naturopathic Medicine in Portland, Oregon. He feels he can be most helpful in cases of infertility that stem from poor endocrine balance, leading to a poor environment for implantation of the embryo. "Pituitary, thyroid, adrenal, and ovarian dysfunctions are usually associated with this picture," he explains. "Pathological uterus, congenitally abnormal reproductive organs—these things are not going to be responsive to what I do." Dr. Russ uses shiatsu massage, craniosacral therapy, and chiropractic with patients for various health problems.

Dr. Russ recalls one thirty-eight-year-old female patient who came to him for neck pain and also mentioned that she was infertile. He told her he might be able to help, but that he couldn't guarantee success. She had stopped working with her fertility specialist and was willing to try anything. "I did chiropractic work on her, full-spine and extremities, and focused on her lumbopelvic region." He stimulated the Chapman's reflexes on the pubic bone and sacrum for the reproductive organs and taught her to stimulate them as well. She also began taking supplements for spleen, ovary, and thyroid. "Most women over thirty-five are at least a little bit hypothyroid, and this affects the ovary and uterus via lack of negative feedback to the pituitary gland," he explains. "She finally conceived about a year later. Whether or not it was because of the work we did, I'll never know, but it was satisfying to see her so happy about it."

CRANIOSACRAL THERAPY

Craniosacral therapy holds promise for dealing with certain kinds of infertility. This therapy is based on the idea that the motion of cranial bones is closely connected to a network of fluids and tissues at the body's core, including the motion of cerebrospinal fluid, the spinal cord, the brain, and the membranes surrounding the central nervous system and sacrum. Craniosacral therapy is a gentle, noninvasive, hands-on approach in which a doctor uses his or her fingers to tune into what's happening in the body.

Dr. Russ explains more thoroughly: "Craniosacral therapy is a technique that originated in the 1970s with an osteopath by the name of John Upledger. His work was based on previous cranial studies by the osteopath Sutherland. Contrary to what anatomists and most physicians are taught, the bones of the cranium move. The movement is slight, rhythmic, and very important to the function of the central nervous system. Rhythmic volume changes in the cerebrospinal fluid are the impulse behind the movement. If the movement is restricted by osseous restriction (in cranial sutures or transitional areas such as occiput/C1) or by dural adhesion, the function of the central nervous system is impaired. Craniosacral therapy techniques are designed to free these restrictions and restore function to the system."

Certain types of movement restriction can impair the function of the central nervous system, Dr. Russ explains. One of these is osseous restriction (in cranial sutures—the joints between the skull bones—or transitional areas). Another is dural adhesion, an abnormal attachment or sticking together of the *dura mater* ("tough mother" in Latin) with other connective tissue around the spine, such as ligaments or fatty tissue. The dura mater is the thick, tough covering around the brain and spinal cord that is continuous with the connective tissue of the nerves leaving the spine. These kinds of adhesions are often the result of injury. "Craniosacral therapy techniques are designed to free these restrictions and restore function to the system," says Dr. Russ.

Doctors use touch to help the body resolve patterns of disorder. Craniosacral therapy can be considered holistic, as it takes the mind, body, and spirit of a patient into account. It is considered effective in treating a broad array of acute and chronic illnesses, including some types of infertility, according to the Craniosacral Therapy Association of North America (CSTA/NA) (www.craniosacraltherapy.org). Though it may sound esoteric, it is more complex than this brief introduction. Think of it as just that—an introduction. Visit the CSTA/NA website to learn more.

THE WURN TECHNIQUE

One exciting, patented form of physical medicine for treating female infertility that has been making headlines is called the WURN Technique. The therapy, a combination of site-specific massage and physical therapy, requires no drugs or surgery. Gentle, highly specific manual pressure is applied over restricted areas, and the therapy treats adhesions and mechanical factors that cause pain and account for about half of all cases of female infertility. Adhesions tend to result from abdominal and gynecologic surgeries, following inflammation associated with bladder or yeast infections, endometriosis or pelvic inflammatory disease, or following trauma, as in tailbone, hip, and back injuries. Adhesions can cause poor functioning of the

A Success Story
Contributed by David Russ, D.C.

I had a thirty-year-old female patient who had low back pain and, incidentally, had not been able to conceive after two years of trying. She was anxious about being adjusted in the usual way, so I used craniosacral work, which is very gentle. It consisted of very light, prolonged application of pressure using contacts and vectors that reintroduced motion and function to the primary craniosacral respiratory system—the subtle but measurable movement of the skull, spine, and pelvis associated with the movement of cerebrospinal fluid. I also prescribed some exercises. The case worked out very well. Her low back pain resolved, she conceived within six months, and she now has a lovely son.

fimbriae (fringed extremities of the Fallopian tubes), blocked Fallopian tubes, restriction of the ovaries, or deviation of the cervix, which makes it hard for sperm to pass through. In addition, the uterine wall's ability to allow implantation of an egg can be impaired by adhesions, causing a miscarriage after fertilization. Decreased hormone function can result when adhesions are on the ovaries, compromising fertility. In terms of female reproductive health, practitioners using the technique report seeing good results with infertility reversal, opening blocked Fallopian tubes, boosting sexual function, improving FSH levels, and alleviating pain associated with menstruation, ovulation, and intercourse.

The goals of treatment are to eliminate pain and restore normal structure, function, and movement. The technique is named after physical therapists Larry and Belinda Wurn, members of the research group in Florida that has received patent protection for it. The overall success rate of reversing fertility among patients who were diagnosed as infertile after two years of not becoming pregnant, who have completed the group's recommended twenty hours of therapy, is 60 to 70 percent. The group in Florida has data showing that, if therapy is unsuccessful, a subsequent IVF will be twice as likely to lead to pregnancy in patients who have first gone through WURN Technique therapy. The technique may help some women avoid costly surgeries that can lead to even more adhesion formation. (Visit www.clearpassage.com for more information about this technique.)

MICROCURRENT THERAPY

Microcurrent therapy relates to the electrical nature of the human body. This therapy delivers minute amounts of electrical stimuli intended to mirror the cellular electrical charges within the body. The microcurrent machine provides a gentle yet powerful form of physical therapy that has been used for over fifteen years. It produces a very small current similar to the body's own current, measured in millionths of an amp. The idea that more is better does not always ring true. After all, in all aspects of life, often a nudge with the right timing and placement is so much more effective than a shove at the wrong time. When applied by a skilled healthcare provider, microcurrent therapy seems to help the body regain a healthier balance. Some practitioners and patients report achieving normal reproductive function and enhanced fertility following microcurrent treatment, though little research has been conducted so far.

Microcurrent frequencies appear to be able to resonate with different biologic tissues and change their structure with the right frequency, balancing organ systems, among other benefits. The idea is that the microcurrent boosts levels of ATP, the body's form of energy, as well as increasing protein synthesis and promoting removal of waste products. It can't be felt during treatment and there is no danger of muscle spasms.

As used in alternative medicine, microcurrent therapy is still very much an investigative tool. And many naturopathic medical schools, for instance, do not train students in microcurrent techniques, though many types of practitioners gain a level of expertise outside of core curriculum in other educational venues. As with all techniques, both proven and not yet supported by scientific literature, keeping expectations within the realm of reasonable is important. Whether it be microcurrent or any other technique, a good dose of common sense can go a long way. However, patients routinely report good results from microcurrent therapy when used for conditions it has been reported to benefit. (It should not be used through a pregnant uterus.)

A Success Story
Contributed by Rosetta Koach, L.M.T., N.D.

I tried for sixteen years to get pregnant. I was married eighteen years ago, and once we stopped doing any prevention, I didn't get pregnant for the next five years, so I started doing a fertility workup and discovered that I had polycystic ovaries. Doctors put me on Clomid, so I took it for two months and began feeling a little crazy on it. I started fighting with my husband—and we never fight—so I stopped it. We ended up going through marriage counseling for the next seven months, and I temporarily stopped thinking about kids. I found an alternative M.D. in California who put me on thyroid medication and had me change my diet, nutrition, and vitamin intake. I started cleaning up allergies and such, but I didn't get pregnant. I took myself off the thyroid medication about a year later. Then we stopped trying to get pregnant because my mom got sick. Her whole dying process, going through the medical establishment, was very traumatic. At some point someone handed me a book on naturopathic medicine, and I went, "Oh my God, this is a better way."

After my mom died, I started learning about naturopathic medicine, and I was accepted into the National College of Naturopathic Medicine (NCNM). I started going through school and healing a lot of illnesses that I'd had (chronic fatigue syndrome and more). Tests revealed that I

GENTLE THERAPIES TREAT THE WHOLE PERSON

It should be clear by now that physical medicine has a lot to offer many infertile couples. In addition to effectively enhancing fertility in many cases, the safe and gentle therapies described here don't pose the risks and potentially dangerous side effects associated with many fertility drugs. They are relatively affordable compared to high-tech surgeries, making them even more appealing as options to consider trying first, or in tandem with other treatments. Refer to the Resources section at the back of this book if you would like more information on the therapies outlined here.

Like other natural therapies covered throughout this book, physical medicine tends to view a person holistically, looking at the whole person when trying to identify health problems and how best to treat them. Preventing problems by living

had hypothyroid, so I was put on thyroid treatment again. I cleaned up my diet really well, started taking vitamins off and on and herbal stuff, homeopathy, TCM, acupuncture, all of it geared toward healing me and getting me pregnant. I also had amennorhea and would only have my menses once a year. Every time I went to M.D.s and told them I wanted to get pregnant, they all wanted to put me on Clomed. They wouldn't talk about anything else related to my health. I wanted to heal my body and get pregnant more naturally.

Going through school I was healing my body, and I went through an enormous amount of healing over the next eight years. About a year after I graduated, my menses were still really irregular—it was the last health thing that I hadn't straightened out. Finally, about a year after I graduated, I went to a workshop about Unda homeopathic products. I tried the Unda female balancing remedies for correcting fertility and menses. Within three weeks I had my first menses. I waited another month, and I had a perfect menses with no problems. After six months I wasn't pregnant yet, but my hormones were really straight. I use a therapy called microcurrent, using microfrequencies for various parts of the body. I had used the microcurrent to heal my thyroid about a year before getting out of school, and my thyroid has been normal ever since. I ran the microcurrent on the ovaries (which had cysts) and that caused me to ovulate. I was pregnant soon after. The baby was born very healthy. Now he's fourteen months, and he's incredible.

healthfully and dealing with the very root of the problem—as opposed to just treating symptoms—is key to these philosophies. Draw on what you've learned here to help make yourselves as healthy and fertile as you can be. Hopefully, one day soon you'll begin passing on your healthy habits to your new baby.

You have just made an investment in your pursuit of the ultimate dream—to become a parent. By now, after reading these pages, you should have gleaned a wealth of useful information about how to enhance your fertility naturally as a couple. Check out the Resources section to learn more or to find a practitioner to help you along. Our hope is that your love for and commitment to your dreams will yield healthier bodies and minds for both of you, so that you may become more fertile while your relationship continues to flourish.

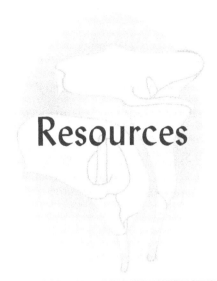

Resources

Infertility

**The American Infertility
  Association (New York, NY)**
www.americaninfertility.org

Fertilinet
www.Fertilinet.com

Fertilitext
www.Fertilitext.org

**The InterNational Council
  on Infertility Information
  Dissemination, Inc. (INCIID)**
www.inciid.org

**RESOLVE: The National Infertility
  Association**
www.resolve.org

Preconception, Prenatal, and Motherhood

BabyCenter
www.babycenter.com

BabyFamily Pregnancy Test
www.BabyFamily.com

Conceiving Concepts, Inc.
www.conceivingconcepts.com

FertileThoughts
www.fertilethoughts.net

**Fertility Institute of New Jersey
  and New York**
www.center4ivf.com

**FertilityPlus (information written
  by patients, for patients)**
www.FertilityPlus.com

Fertility UK
www.FertilityUK.org

**Onna.org (search engine for
  prenatal and fertility websites)**
www.onna.org

**Pacific Gynecology Specialists
  (Seattle, Washington)**
Tel.: 206-215-3200

ParentsPlace.com
www.parentsplace.com/fertility

Preconception.com
www.Preconception.com

TTC Int'l, LLC
www.TryingToConceive.com

Miscarriage Resources

Born Angels Pregnancy Loss Support
www.bornangels.com/

Pregnancyloss.info
www.pregnancyloss.info/

**FertilityPlus Miscarriage Support &
Information Resources**
www.fertilityplus.org/faq/miscarriage/
resources.html

Tefilat Chana
www.chanasprayer.org

Books on Infertility

Berger, Gary S., Marc Goldstein, and Mark Fuerst. 1989. *The Couple's Guide to Fertility.* New York, NY: Main Street Books, 1995. (Extra focus on assisted reproduction techniques)

Barbieri, Robert L., M.D., editor, et al. *Six Steps to Increased Fertility: An Integrated Medical and Mind/Body Program To Promote Conception.* New York, NY: Simon & Schuster, 2000.

Boland, Katie. *I Got Pregnant, You Can Too!: How Healing Yourself Physically, Mentally, and Spiritually Leads to Fertility.* Grass Valley, CA: Underwood Books, 1998.

Domar, Alice D. and Henry Dreher. *Healing Mind, Healthy Woman: Using the Mind-Body Connection to Manage Stress and Take Control of Your Life.* New York, NY: Henry Holt, 1996.

Edwards, Margot. *A Stairstep Approach to Fertility.* Freedom, CA: Crossing Press, 1989.

Indichova, Julia. *Inconceivable: Winning the Fertility Game.* New York, NY: Adell Press, 1997.

Liebmann-Smith, Joan, et al. *The Unofficial Guide to Overcoming Infertility.* New York, NY: Hungry Minds, Inc., 1998.

Parvati, Jeannine, et al. *Conscious Conception.* Joseph, UT: Freestone Publishing, 1986.

Reiss, Fern. *The Infertility Diet: Get Pregnant and Prevent Miscarriage.* Newton, MA: Peanut Butter and Jelly Press, 1999.

Shannon, Marilyn M. *Fertility, Cycles, and Nutrition.* Cincinnati, OH: Couple to Couple League International, 2001.

Weschler, Toni. *Taking Charge of Your Fertility*. New York, NY: HarperCollins, 2002.

Williams, Christopher, M.D. *The Fastest Way To Get Pregnant Naturally*. New York, NY: Hyperion, 2001.

Natural Medicine

Hudson, Tori. *Women's Encyclopedia of Natural Medicine*. Los Angeles, CA: Lowell House, 1999.

Nutrition Resources

Balch, J.F., and P. Balch. *Prescription for Nutritional Healing*. Third edition. New York, NY: Avery/Penguin Putnam, 2000.

Challem, Jack, and Liz Brown. *Basic Health Publications User's Guide to Vitamins and Minerals*. North Bergen, NJ: Basic Health Publications, Inc., 2002.

Marz, Russell B. *Medical Nutrition from Marz*. Portland, OR: Quiet Lion Press, 1999.

Murray, Michael T. *The Healing Power of Foods: Nutrition Secrets for Vibrant Health and Long Life*. Rocklin, CA: Prima Publishing, 1993.

The American Association of Naturopathic Physicians
www.naturopathic.org

Home Food Allergy Test—Available through Health Dynamics
www.myhealthdynamics.com • Tel: 503-430-1307

Environmental Medicine

The American College of Occupational and Environmental Medicine
www.acoem.org

Consumer Product Safety Commission
1-800-638-CPSC

The Environmental Protection Agency (EPA) • www.epa.gov

- For state-approved laboratories, go to www.epa.gov/safewater/faq/sco.html
- To order the EPA's pamphlet on home water filters, call the Environmental Resource Information Center at 1-800-276-0462 and ask for document #R-091.
- For information on air quality, visit www.epa.gov.
- EPA Drinking Water Hotline: 1-800-426-4791

NSF International

www.nsf.org • Tel: 1-800-673-8010

The Water Quality Association

www.wqa.org (offers a list of approved units for removing contaminants)
   Tel: 708-505-0160

www.waterqualityreports.org (an excellent resource for water-quality
   information)

TCM-Related Resources

American Association of Oriental Medicine (AAOM)

www.aaom.org • Tel.: 610-266-1433

Molony, David. *The American Association of Oriental Medicine's Complete Guide
to Chinese Herbal Medicine: How to Treat Illness and Maintain Wellness with Chinese Herbs.* New York, NY: The Berkley Publishing Group, 1998.

National Certification Commission for Acupuncture and Oriental Medicine

nccaom.org

Vital Age International, Inc.

P.O. Box 5506
105 Lewis St., Suite 207
Ketchum, ID 83340
www.VitalAge.com • Tel: 208-727-0077 / Fax: 208-727-0066

Homeopathic Medicine

To Find a Homeopath in Your Area

www.homeopathyhome.com/directory/usa/organisations.shtml

www.homeopathic.org/find.htm

www.healthy.net/clinic/refer/HomeopathySearchIndex.asp

www.nccn.net/~wwithin/STEVELIST.htm

Homeopathic Pharmacies

Hahnemann Laboratories, Inc.

www.hahnemannlabs.com

Helios Homoeopathic Pharmacy
www.helios.co.uk

Homeopathy Home Listing of U.S. Homeopathic Pharmacies
www.homeopathyhome.com/directory/usa/pharmacies.shtml

National Center for Homeopathy (NCH)
www.homeopathic.org

Homeopathy Books

Jonas, Wayne B., Jennifer Jacobs. *Healing With Homeopathy.* New York, NY: Warner Books, Inc., 1996.

Ullman, Dana. *The Consumer's Guide to Homeopathy.* New York, NY: G.P. Putnam's Sons, 1995.

Physical Medicine

The American Chiropractic Association (ACA)
www.amerchiro.org

The Craniosacral Therapy Association of North America (CSTA/NA)
www.craniosacraltherapy.org

The International College of Applied Kinesiology (ICAK)
www.icakusa.com

The WURN Technique
www.clearpassage.com

Supplements: Research and Journal Abstracts

Fertil Male Supplement from Lane Labs
www.lanelabs.com/fertilmale/

MEDLINE
www.ncbi.nlm.nih.gov/entrez/query

National Center for Complementary and Alternative Medicine,
   National Institutes of Health (NIH)
nccam.nih.gov/nccam

Glossary

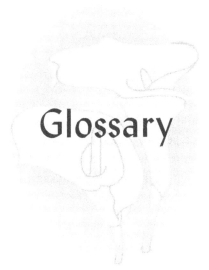

acid a substance that dissociates into one or more hydrogen ions and one or more anions, or negative ions. Acids are proton donors.

acrosome a dense granule in the head of sperm that contains enzymes to aid the sperm in penetrating an ovum (egg), or secondary oocyte.

acupressure a Chinese healing therapy that stimulates energy and relieves symptoms with massage and hand-and-finger pressure on meridian points and channels on the skin.

acupuncture a Chinese healing therapy in which thin, sterile needles are inserted into the skin at specific meridian points along the body to stimulate energy, encouraging balance of hormone function and organ interaction and to provide pain relief.

antioxidants nutrient and plant substances that help combat free radicals and protect the body.

asbestosis a lung disease caused by asbestos.

asthenospermia reduced sperm motility in semen.

azoospermia the complete absence of living sperm in semen.

base a substance that dissociates into one or more hydroxide ions or one or more cations, or positive ions. Bases are proton acceptors.

cholesterol a naturally occurring substance in all animals, including humans. It is an essential building block for steroid hormones in the body including sex hormones and vitamin D, but high levels can lead to health problems, including heart disease.

chorion the outer membrane surrounding the fetus that attaches to the uterus, makes the hormone hCG, and later becomes the placenta.

corpus luteum the mature ovarian follicle in females that ruptures to expel a potential mature ovum, or egg.

diabetes the most common form is called type 2 diabetes and is generally not insulin dependent, whereas type 1 is typically called insulin-dependent diabetes. Diabetes is a health condition that results from the inability of the body to properly use blood sugar (glucose), resulting in elevated blood sugar levels when not properly treated.

DHA an essential fatty acid critical for neurological development, especially in developing unborn babies and in early child development.

DNA the body's genetic material.

dysmenorrhea difficult and often painful menstruation.

EPA an essential fatty acid, that possesses many properties including fueling the anti-inflammatory and pro-immune pathways within the body.

endometrium the mucous membrane that lines the uterus.

epididymis comma-shaped male organ that lies along the posterior border of the testis and contains the ductus epididymis, where sperm undergo maturation.

essential fatty acids (EFAs) fatty acids not produced in the body and, therefore, must be obtained in the diet.

estradiol the most potent of the three major forms of estrogen in the body.

estrogen the hormone most frequently called the "female hormone," though it is present in both men and women, it is associated most strongly with the sex characteristics of females.

exogenous estrogens these forms of estrogen are produced from sources external to the body, and thus are "ex-tra" burdens to the body.

follicle the beginning site for the formation of the ovum, or egg.

free radicals substances that the body is exposed to that cause oxidative damage, and require antioxidants to quench.

gametes the representative portions of either the male or female DNA contribution to conception.

gestational diabetes a form of diabetes that sometimes occurs during pregnancy.

HDL known as the "good cholesterol," high-density lipoproteins help prevent plaque buildup in the arteries.

hyperkalemia higher-than-normal blood levels of potassium, which can lead to muscle weakness, diarrhea, and heart problems related to changes in electrical impulse.

hypokalemia lower-than-normal blood levels of potassium, which can lead to muscle weakness, heart arrhythmias, breathing problems, nausea, and other conditions.

hysterosalpingogram an exam involving an x-ray of the uterus and Fallopian tubes after the injection of a special dye through the cervix.

idiopathic oligospermia unexplained low sperm count.

infertility when a couple at a given point in time has not been able to conceive after a year of active intercourse.

LDL the proverbial "bad cholesterol," low-density lipoproteins are linked to cardiovascular disease.

laparoscopy an outpatient surgical procedure in which the pelvis is examined through a small incision in the navel.

lipid peroxidation arises from free-radical damage either due to chemical, light, or heat exposure of fatty substances including cholesterol.

luteal phase the phase of the menstrual cycle following ovulation, during which the corpus luteum makes progesterone that causes the uterine lining to make substances that support the early embryo in implantation and growth.

luteinizing hormone (LH) a hormone produced by the pituitary gland in the brain that is involved in the development of the corpus luteum.

miscarriage when there is an unintentional loss of a developing baby.

mitochondria cell structures often referred to as the "powerhouses" of cells due to their role in energy production.

monounsaturated fat a form of fat found in olive oil and nuts that possesses only a single "mono" unsaturated chemical bond.

motility the ability of the sperm to move forward toward the egg.

moxibustion a therapy used in Chinese medicine that entails the burning of moxa, dried mugwort, to produce heat and warm the body to activate the Qi.

neonatal the first four weeks after birth.

oocyte an immature egg.

oligoasthenospemia low seminal secretion and reduced sperm motility.

oligospermia having scanty seminal secretion.

ovulation when the egg is released.

ovum an egg.

PCBs polychlorinated biphenyls, potentially linked to deteriorating sperm quality and quantity.

phytoestrogens simple plant-based chemicals that have estrogenlike effects within the body.

polyunsaturated fats fats that possess more than one unsaturated chemical body.

postovulatory phase the portion of a woman's menstrual cycle that occurs after ovulation.

preovulatory the portion of a woman's menstrual cycle that occurs prior to ovulation.

progesterone the hormone that basically helps balance out estrogen and serves to maintain a pregnancy and the uterine lining.

prostatitis inflammation of the prostate gland.

Qi (pronounced "chee") the vital essence of life found in all living things, according to traditional Chinese medicine.

RNA ribonucleic acid relays instructions from genes to guide the assembly of amino acids into proteins in each cell.

reproductive endocrinologist a specialist in the evaluation and treatment of infertility.

saturated fat those fats in which all the chemical bonds are saturated and which are typically either man-made or from animal sources.

secondary infertility infertility in which there has been a previous pregnancy.

semen a mixture of sperm and secretions of the prostate gland, bulbourethral glands, and seminal vesicles that is ejaculated.

seminal plasmin an antibiotic in semen that can destroy bacteria in semen and in the female reproductive tract that has the potential to hinder fertilization.

sperm motility a term that reflects the ability of sperm to move appropriately.

spermatogenesis the formation and development of sperm that occurs in the seminiferous tubules of the testes.

stratum functionalis the inner endometrium layer next to the uterine cavity that makes up the maternal part of the placenta during pregnancy and is shed during menstruation.

superovulation the release of two or more eggs.

teratogenic capable of causing malformation of a developing baby.

testosterone the main male sex hormone, responsible for male sex organs, secondary sexual characteristics, sperm, and body growth. Women also produce small amounts.

trans-fatty acids classically created from the heating of oils, such a frying or other such cooking or food processing. Trans fats are deleterious to one's health.

varicoceles varicose veins in the scrotum and the most common cause of male infertility.

vas deferens tubes that carry testicular fluid and sperm to the ejaculatory ducts.

vasoepididymostomy a procedure connecting the vas deferens to the epididymis in order to reverse a vasectomy with epididymal obstruction.

VOCs volatile organic compounds are compounds that can be expelled from the materials containing them and released into the air, which can lead to sinus and lung irritation.

xenoestrogens estrogenlike compounds that come from outside the body and mimic estrogens once in the body.

zygote a single-celled fertilized ovum, or egg.

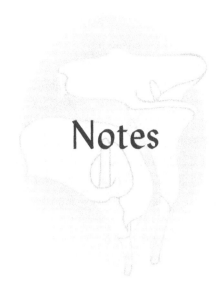

Notes

Chapter 1

1. RJ Aitken, "The role of free oxygen radicals and sperm function," *Int J Androl* 1989;12:95–97.

2. SA Suleiman, ME Ali, ZM Zaki, et al., "Lipid peroxidation and human sperm motility: protective role of vitamin E," *J Androl* 1996;17(5):530–537.

3. K Dabrowski, A Ciereszko, "Ascorbic acid protects against male infertility in a teleost fish," *Experientia* 1996;52(2):97–100.

4. BK Petroff, RE Ciereszko, K Dabrowski, et al., "Depletion of vitamin C from pig corpora lutea by prostaglandin F2 alpha-induced secretion of the vitamin," *J Reprod Fertil* 1998;112(2):243–247.

5. J Tarin, J Ten , FJ Vendrell, et al., "Effects of maternal ageing and dietary antioxidant supplementation on ovulation, fertilisation and embryo development in vitro in the mouse," *Reprod Nutr Dev* 1998;38(5):499–508.

6. WY Wong, CM Thomas, JM Merkus, et al., "Male factor subfertility: possible causes and the impact of nutritional factors," *Fertil Steril* 2000;73(3):435–442.

7. A Favier, "[Current aspects about the role of zinc in nutrition]," *Rev Prat* 1993;43(2):146–151.

8. CM Bulik, PF Sullivan, JL Fear, et al., "Fertility and reproduction in women with anorexia nervosa: a controlled study," *J Clin Psychiatry* 1999;60(2):130–135.

9. C Galletly, A Clark, L Tomlinson, et al., "A group program for obese, infertile women: weight loss and improved psychological health," *J Psychosom Obstet Gynaecol* 1996;17(2):125–128.

10. E Weisberg, "Smoking and reproductive health," *Clin Reprod Fertil* 1985;3(3):175–186.

11. R Rozati, PP Reddy, P Reddanna, et al., "Xenoestrogens and male infertility: myth or reality?" *Asian J Androl* 2000;2(4):263–269.

12. GM Buck, JE Vena, EF Schisterman, et al., "Parental consumption of contaminated sport fish from Lake Ontario and predicted fecundability," *Epidem* 2000;11(4):388–393.

13. WH Kutteh, CH Chao, JO Ritter, et al., "Vaginal lubricants for the infertile couple: effect on sperm activity," *Intl Jour of Fert & Men Studies* 1996;41(4):400–404.

14. Z Zheng, "Analysis on the therapeutic effect of combined use of acupuncture and meditation in 297 cases of male sterility," *J Tradit Chin Med* 1997;17(3):190–193.

15. Y Zhai, L Xu , F Xu, et al., "TCM treatment of male infertility due to seminal abnormality—a clinical observation of 82 cases," *J Tradit Chin Med* 1990;10(1):26–29.

16. F Lian, "TCM treatment of luteal phase defect—an analysis of 60 cases," *J Tradit Chin Med* 1991;11(2):115–120.

17. G Salvati, G Genovesi, L Marcellini, et al., "Effects of Panax Ginseng C.A. Meyer saponins on male fertility," *Panminerva Medica* 1996;38(4):249–254.

Chapter 2

1. BB Green, NS Weiss, JR Daling, "Risk of ovulatory infertility in relation to body weight," *Fertil Steril* 1988;50(5):721–726.

2. DE Stewart, E Robinson, DS Goldbloom, "Infertility and eating disorders," *Am J Obstet Gynecol* 1990;163(5 Pt 1):1196–1199.

3. CM Bulik, PF Sullivan, et al., "Fertility and reproduction in women with anorexia nervosa: a controlled study," *J Clin Psychiatry* 1999;60(2):130–135.

4. SJ Crow, P Thuras, et al., "Long-term menstrual and reproductive function in patients with bulimia nervosa," *Am J Psychiatry* 2002;159(6):1048–1050.

5. BC Bowles, BP Williamson, "Pregnancy and lactation following anorexia and bulimia," *J Obstet Gynecol Neonatal Nurs* 1990;19(3):243–248.

6. RE Frisch, "Body fat, menarche, fitness and fertility," *Hum Reprod* 1987;2(6): 521–533.

7. Melvyn R Werbach with Jeffrey Moss, *Textbook of Nutritional Medicine* (Tarzana, CA: Third Line Press, Inc., 1999).

8. F Grodstein, MB Goldman, DW Cramer, "Infertility in women and moderate alcohol use," *Am J Public Health* 1994;84(9):1429–1432.

9. MR Luck, I Jeyaseelan, RA Scholes, "Ascorbic acid and fertility," *Biol Reprod* 1995; 52(2):262–266.

10. BK Petroff, RE Ciereszko, et al., "Depletion of vitamin C from pig corpora lutea by prostaglandin F2 alpha-induced secretion of the vitamin," *J Reprod Fertil* 1998;112(2): 243–247.

11. J Tarin, J Ten, FJ Vendrell, et al., "Effect of maternal ageing and dietary antioxidant supplementation on ovulation, fertilization and embryo development in vitro in the mouse," *Reprod Nutr Dev* 1998;38(5):499–508.

12. M Tikkiwal, RL Ajmera, NK Mathur, "Effect of zinc administration on seminal zinc and fertility of oligospermic males," *Indian J Physiol Pharmacol* 1987;31(1):30–34.

13. SA Suleiman, ME Ali, et al., "Lipid peroxidation and human sperm motility: protective role of vitamin E," *J Androl* 1996;17(5):530–537.

14. C Battalia, M Salvatori, et al., "Adjuvant L-arginine treatment of in-vitro fertilization in poor responder patients," *Hum Reprod* 1999;14(7):1690–1697.

15. D De Aloysio, et al., "The clinical use of arginine aspartate in male infertility," *Acta Eur fertile* 1982;13(3):133–167.

16. A Schachter, et al., "Treatment of oligospermia with the amino acid arginine," *J Urol* 1973;110(3):311–313.

17. C Jeulin, LM Lewin, "Role of free L-carnitine and acetyl-L-carnitine in post-gonadal maturation of mammalian spermatozoa," *Hum Reprod Update* 1996;2(2): 87–102.

18. F Mazzilli, T Rossi, et al., "[Intra-spermatic L-carnitine and survival of sperm motility]," *Minerva Ginecol* 1999;51(4):129–134.

19. M Costa, D Canale, et al., "L-carnitine in idiopathic asthenospermia: a multicenter study," *Andrologia* 1994;26(3):155–159.

20. R Scott, A MacPherson, et al., "The effect of oral selenium supplementation on human sperm motility," *Br J Urol* 1998;82(1):76–80.

21. B Sandler, et al., "Treatment of oligospermia with vitamin B_{12}," *Infertility* 1984;7: 133–138.

22. A Mancini, G Conte, et al., "Relationship between sperm cell ubiquinone and seminal parameters in subjects with and without varicocele," *Andrologia* 1998;30(1):1–4.

23. A Lewin, H Lavon, "The effect of coenzyme Q_{10} on sperm motility and function," *Mol Aspects Med* 1997;18 suppl:S213–S219.

24. AE Czeizel, "Periconceptional folic acid containing multivitamin supplementation," *Eur J Obstet Gynecol Reprod Biol* 1998;78(2):151–161.

25. TO Scholl, TP Stein, "Oxidant damage to DNA and pregnancy outcome," *J Matern Fetal Med* 2001;10(3):182–185.

26. L Multigner, A Oliva, "Secular variations in sperm quality: fact or science fiction?" *Cad Saude Publica* 2002;Mar–Apr, 18(2):403–12.

27. JW Dallinga, EJ Moonen, et al., "Decreased human semen quality and organochlorine compounds in blood," *Hum Reprod* 2002;17(8):1973–1979.

28. R Rozati, PP Reddy, et al., "Xenoestrogens and male infertility: myth or reality?" *Asian J Androl* 2000;2(4):263–269.

29. PJ Sauer, M Huisman, et al., "Effects of polychlorinated biphenyls (PCBs) and dioxins on growth and development," *Hum Exp Toxicol* 1994;13(12):900–906.

30. GM Buck, LE Sever, et al., "Consumption of contaminated sport fish from Lake Ontario and time-to-pregnancy," *Am J Epidemiol* 1997;146(11):949–954.

31. C Charlier, G Plomteux, "[Endocrine disruption and organochlorine pesticides]," *Acta Clin Belg Suppl* 2002;1:2–7.

32. B Xu, SE Chia, M Tsakok, et al., "Trace elements in blood and seminal plasma and their relationship to sperm quality," *Reprod Toxicol* 1993;7:613–618.

33. C Winder, "Lead, reproduction and development," *Neurotoxicology* 1993;14(2–3): 303–317.

34. David Steinman and Samuel Epstein, *The Safe Shopper's Bible* (New York, NY: Hungry Minds, Inc., 1995).

35. John Bower, *The Healthy House: How to Buy One, How to Build One, How to Cure a Sick One*, IV (Bloomington, IN: The Healthy House Institute, 2001).

36. WH Kutteh, CH Chao, et al., "Vaginal lubricants for the infertile couple: effect on sperm activity," *Human Reprod* 1998;13(12):3351–3356.

Chapter 3

1. A Zdziennicki, T Laudanski, "[Iron deficiency as a risk factor during the perinatal period]," *Ginekol Pol* 1996;67(6):301–303.

2. DG Kramer, ST Brown, "Sexually transmitted diseases and infertility," *Int J Gynaecol Obstet* 1984;22(1):19–27.

Chapter 4

1. Federation CECOS, D Schwartz, JM Mayaux, "Female fecundity as a function of age: results of artificial insemination in 2,193 nulliparous women with azoospermic husbands," *N Engl J Med* 1982; 306:404.

2. F Bolumar, J Olsen, M Rebagliato, et al., "Caffeine intake and delayed conception: a European multicenter study on infertility and subfecundity. European Study Group on Infertility Subfecundity," *Am J Epidemiol* 1997;145(4):324–334.

3. E de la Rochebrochard, P Thonneau, "Paternal age and maternal age are risk factors for miscarriage; results of a multicentre European study," *Hum Reprod* 2002;17(6):1649–1656.

4. SA Kidd, B Eskenazi, AJ Wyrobek, "Effects of male age on semen quality and fertility: A review of the literature," *Fertil Steril* 2001;75(2):237–248.

5. M Munafo, M Murphy, D Whiteman, et al., "Does cigarette smoking increase time to conception?" *J Biosoc Sci* 2002;34(1):65–73.

6. AJ Wilcox, CR Weinberg, DD Baird, "Timing of sexual intercourse in relation to ovulation: Effects on the probability of conception, survival of the pregnancy, and sex of the baby," *N Engl J Med* 1995;333:1517–1521.

Chapter 6

1. M Sigman, LI Lipshultz, SS Howards, "Evaluation of the subfertile male" in *Infertility in the Male*, 3rd edition (St. Louis, MO: Mosby, 1997), 173–193.

2. J Jarow, "Effects of varicocele in male fertility," *Hum Reprod* 2001;7(update no.1):59–64.

3. I Madgar, R Weissenberg, et al., "Controlled trial of high spermatic vein ligation for varicocele in infertile men," *Fertil Steril* 1995;63:120–124.

4. E Nieschlag, L Hertle, A Fischedick, "Update on treatment of varicocle: counseling as effective as occlusion of the vena spermatica," *Hum Reprod* 1998;13:2147–2150.

5. AM Belker, AJ Thomas Jr., et al., "Results of 1,469 microsurgical vasectomy reversals by the Vasovasostomy Study Group," *J Urol* 1991;145:505–511.

6. EF Fuch, R Burt, "Vasectomy reversal performed 15 years or more after vasectomy: correlation of pregnancy outcome with partner age and with pregnancy results of *in vitro* fertilization with intracytoplasmic sperm injection," *Fertil Steril* 2002;77:516–519.

7. MT Murray, "Male infertility: A growing concern," *Am J Natural Med,* 4(3):6–19.

Chapter 8

1. GD Premalatha, J Ravindran, "Reproductive problems of the work force," *Med J Malaysia* 2000;55(2):146–151.

2. F Grodstein, MB Goldman, et al., "Infertility in women and moderate alcohol use," *Am J Public Health* 1994;84:1429–1432.

3. G Howe, C Westhoff, M Vessey, et al., "Effects of age, cigarette smoking, and other factors on fertility. Findings in a large prospective study," *BMJ* 1985;290:1697–1699.

4. CR Weinberg, AJ Wilcox, et al., "Reduced fecundability in women with prenatal exposure to cigarette smoking," *Am J Epidemiol* 1989;129:1072–1078.

5. E Weisberg, "Smoking and reproductive health," *Clin Reprod Fertil* 1985;3:175–186.

6. T Ochedalski, A Lachowicz-Ochedalska et al., "Examining the effects of tobacco smoking on levels of certain hormones in serum of young men," *Ginekol Pol* 1994;65:87–93.

7. NB Oldereid, Y Thomassen, et al., "Seminal plasma lead, cadmium, and zinc in relation to tobacco consumption," *Int J Androl* 1994:17:24–28.

8. F Grodstein, MB Goldman, L Ryan, DW Cramer, "Relation of female infertility consumption of caffeinated beverages," *Am J Epidemiol* 1993;137:1353–1360.

9. EE Hatch, MB Bracken, "Association of delayed conception with caffeine consumption," *Am J Epidemiol* 1993;138:1082–1092.

10. CK Stanton, RH Gray, "Effects of caffeine consumption on delayed conception," *Am J Epidemiol* 1995;142:1322–1329.

11. L Fenster, A Bubbard, G Windhan, R Hiatt, et al., "A prospective study of caffeine consumption and spontaneous abortion," *Am J Epidemiol* 1996;143(11):525.

12. DW Cramer, Letter, *Lancet* 1990;33:792.

13. M Wynn, A Wynn, "Slimming and fertility," *Mod Midwife* Jun 1994;4(6):17–20.

14. RM Sharpe, "The 'oestrogen hypothesis': Where do we stand now?" *Int J Androl* 2003;26(1):2–15.

15. S Sinclair, "Male fertility: Nutritional and environmental considerations," *Altern Med Rev* 2000;5(1):28–38.

16. R Rozati, PP Reddy, P Reddanna, R Mujtaba, "Xenoesterogens and male infertility: myth or reality?" *Asian J Androl* 2000;2(4):263–269.

17. MD Dickman, KM Leung, "Mercury and organochlorine exposure from fish consumption in Hong Kong," *Chemosphere* 1998;(5):991–1015.

18. GM Buck, JE Vena, et al., "Parental consumption of contaminated sport fish from Lake Onatrio and predicted fecundability," *Epidemiol* 2000;11(4):388–393.

19. DC James, "Eating disorders, fertility, and pregnancy: relationships and complications," *J Perinat Neonatal Nurs* 2001;15(2):36–48.

20. CM Bulik, PF Sullivan, JL Fear, A Pickering, A Dawn, M McCullin, Fertility and reproduction in women with anorexia nervosa: A controlled study," *J Clin Psychilatry* 1999;60(2):130–135.

21. MR Werbach, "Female infertility," *Townsend Letter for Doctors and Patients* 1995;Aug:34 Review.

22. EK Sheiner, E Sheiner, R Carel, et al., "Potential association between male infertility and occupational psychological stress," *J Occup Environ Med* 2002;44(12):1093–9.

23. RF Moseman, "Chemical disposition of boron in animals and humans," *Environ Health Perspect* 1994;102:113–117.

24. DH Rushton, ID Ramsay, JJH Gilkes, "Ferritin and fertility," *Lancet* 1991;337:1554.

25. AE Czeisel, J Metneki, I Dudas, "The effect of preconceptional multivitamin supplementation on fertility," *Internal J Vit Nutr Res* 1996;66:55–58.

26. RH Fletcher, KM Fairfield, "Vitamins for chronic disease prevention in adults: clinical applications," *JAMA* 2002;207(23):3127–3129.

27. M Igarashi, "Augmentative effect of ascorbic acid upon induction of human ovulation in clomiphene-ineffective anovulatory women," *Int J Fertil* 1977;22:168–173.

28. R Bayer, "Treatment of infertility with vitamin E," *Int J Fertil* 1960;5:70–78.

29. E Griffen, Wilson D, "Disorders of the Testes" in *Harrison's Principles of Internal Medicine,* 13th ed. (New York, NY: McGraw-Hill 1994), 2006–2017.

30. K Purvis, E Christiansen, "Male infertility: Current concepts," *Ann Med* 1992;24: 258–272.

31. CG Fraga, PA Motchnik, MK Shigenaga, et al., "Ascorbic acid protects against endogenous oxidative DNA damage in human sperm," *Proc Natl Acad Sci* 1991;88:11003–11006.

32. DP Weller, JS Zaneweld, NR Farnsworth, "Gossypol: Pharmacology and current status as a male contraceptive," *Econ Med Plant Res* 1985;1:87–112.

33. A Lewin, H Lavon, "The effect of coenzyme Q_{10} on sperm motility and function," *Mol Aspect Med* 1997;18:213–219.

34. R Isoyama, S Kawai, et al., "Clinical experience with methylcobalamin in the treatment of oligospermia results of double-blind comparative clinical study," *Hinyokiki Kiyo* 1988;34:1109–1132.

35. B Sandler, B Faragher, "Treatment of oligospermia with vitamin B$_{12}$," *Infertility* 1984;7:133–138.

36. EB Dawson, Harris, et al., "Effect of ascorbic acid on male fertility," *Ann NY Acad Sci* 1987;49:312–323.

37. D Vezina, F Mauffette, KD Roberts, et al., "Selenium-vitamin E supplementation in infertile men. Effects on semen parameters and micronutrient levels and distribution," *Biol Trac Elem Res* 1996;53:65–83.

38. A Netter, R Hartoma, K Nahoul, "Effect of zinc administration on plasma testosterone, dihydrotestosterone and sperm count," *Arch Androl* 1981;7:69–73.

39. M Tikkiwal, RL Ajmera, et al., "Efffect of zinc administration of seminal zinc and fertility of oligospermic males," *Indian J Physiol Pharmacol* 1987;31:30–34.

40. A Schacter, JA Goldman, et al., "Treatment of oligospermia with the amino acid arginine," *J Urol* 1973;110:311–313.

41. M Scibona, P Meschini, et al., "L-arginine and male infertility," *Minerva Urol Nefol* 1994;46:251–253.

42. KL Goa, RN Brodgen, "L-carnitine: A preliminary review of its pharmacokinetics and its therapeutic use in ischemic cardiac disease and primary and secondary deficiencies in relationship to essential fatty acid metabolism," *Drugs* 1987;34:1–24.

43. GF Menchini-Fabris, D Canale, et al., "Free L-carnitine in human semen: Its variability in different andrologic pathologies," *Fertil Steril* 1984;42:263–267.

44. G Vitali, R Parene, et al., "Carnitine supplementation in human idiopathic asthenospermia: Clinical results," *Drugs Exp Clin Res* 1995;21:157–159.

45. R Scott, A MacPheroson, RW Yates, et al., "The effect of oral selenium on human sperm motility," *Br J Urol* 1998;82:76–80.

46. SA Suleiman, ME Ali, ZM Zaki, et al., "Lipid peroxidation and human sperm motility. Protective role of vitamin E," *J Androl* 1996;17:530–537.

47. IN Ibeh, N Uriah, JI Ogonar, "Dietary exposure to aflatoxin in human male infertility in Benin City, Nigeria," *Int J Fertil Menopausal Stud* 1994;39(4):208–214

Chapter 9

1. HY Zhang, XZ Yu, GL Wang, "[Preliminary report of the treatment of luteal phase defect by replenishing kidney. An analysis of 53 cases]," *Zhongguo Zhong XI Yi Jie He Za Zhi* 12(8):473–474.

2. A Milewicz, E Gejedel, H Sworen, et al., "[Vitex agnus castus extract in the treatment of

luteal phase defects due to latent hyperprolactinemia. Results of a randomized placebo-controlled double blind study]," *Arzneimittelforschung* 1993;43(7):752–756.

3. RH Bubenzer, "[Therapy with Agnus castus extract (Strotan(r))]," *Therapiewoche* 1993;43:32–3, 1705–1706.

4. S Usuki, Y Usuki, "Hachimijiogan treatment is effective in the management of infertile women with hyperporlactinemia or bromocriptine-resistant hyperprolactinemia," *Am J Chin Med* 1989;17(3–4):225–241.

5. I Gerhard, A Patek, B Monga, et al., "Mastodyonon [for female sterility]," *Forsch Komplementarmed* 1998;5(6):272–278.

6. DJ Li, CJ Li, Y Zhu, "[Treatments of immunological infertility with Chinese medicinal herbs of ziyin jianghuo]," *Chung Kuo Chung His I Chieh Ho Tsa Chih* 1995;15(1):3–5.

7. T Yaginuma, R Izumi, H Yasui, et al., "[Effect of traditional herbal medicine on serum testosterone levels and its induction of regular ovulation in hyperandrogenic and oligomenorrheic women]," *Nippon Sanka Fujinka Gakki Zasshi* 1982;34(7):939–944.

8. P Tabakova, et al., Clinical study of Tribestan(r) in females with endocrine sterility, as referenced in MR Werbach and MT Murray, *Botanical Influences on Illness* 2nd ed. (Tarzana, CA: Third Line Press Inc., 2000), 399.

9. TK Jensen, TB Henricksen, NH Hjolland, et al., "Caffeine intake and fecundability: A follow-up study among 430 Danish couples planning their first pregnancy," *Reprod Toxicol* 1998;12(3):289–295.

10. K-J Bohnert, "The use of Vitex agnus castus for hyperprolactinemia," *Quarterly Review of Natural Medicine* Spring 1997:19–21

11. J Waynberg, "Aphrodisiacs: Contribution to the clinical validation of the traditional use of Ptychopetalum." Presented at the First International Congress on Ethnopharmacology, Strasbourg, France, June, 1990.

12. G Salvati, G Genovesi, L Marcellini, et al., "Effect of Panax ginseng C.A. Meyer saponins on male fertility," *Panminerva Med* 1996; 38(4):249–254.

13. T Suzkuki, K Kurokawa, et al., "[Clinical effect of Cernilton in chronic prostatitis]," *Hinyokika Kiyo* 1992;38(4):484–494.

14. A Clavert, Cranz, JP Riffaud, et al., "Effects of an extract of the bark of Pygeum africanum (V.1326) on prostatic secretions in the rat and in man," *Ann Urol* 1986;20(5):341–343.

15. C Carnini, V Salvioli, A Scuteri, et al., "Urological and sexual evaluation of treatment of benign prostatic disease using Pygeum africanum at high doses," *J Arch Ital Urol Nefrol Androl* 1991;63(3):341–345.

16. TJ Wilt, et al., "Saw palmetto extracts for treatment of benign prostatic hyperplasia—A systemic review," *JAMA* 1998; 280:1604–1609.

17. GP Yue, Q Chen, N Dai, "[Eighty-seven cases of male infertility treated with Bushen

Shengjing Pill in clinical observation and evaluation on its curative effect]," *Chung Kuo Chung His I Chieh Ho Tsa Chih* 1996;16(8):463–466, 1996.

18. XD Liu, "[Effect of Chinese medicinal herbs on sperm membrane of infertile male]," *Zhong Xi Yi Jie He Za Zhi* 1990;10(9):519–521.

19. CY Hong, J Ku, P Wu, "Astragalus membranaceus stimulates human sperm motility in vitro," *Am J Chin Med* 1992;20(3–4):289–294.

20. RL Zheng, H Zhang, "Effects of ferulic acid on fertile and asthenozoospermic infertile human sperm motlility, viability, lipid peroxidation and cyclic nucleotides," *Free Radic Biol Med* 1997;22(4):581–586.

21. XF Yang, T Wei, J Tong, "[Clinical and experimental study on Composite Wuzi Dihuang Liquor in treating male infertility]," *Chung Kuo Chung His I Chieh Ho Tsa Chih* 1995;15(4):209–212.

22. T Tanifuji, "[Clinical experience of Hachimijiogan for male infertility patients]," *Hinyokika Kiyo* 1984;30(1):97–102.

23. H Yoshida, T Tanifuji, H Sakurai, et al., "[Clinical effects of Chinese herb medicine Hochu-ekki-to on infertile men]," *Hinyokika Kiyo* 1986;32(2):297–302.

24. D Tsetkoc, M Karapandov, M Taskov, "Effect on some forms of male infertility," *Med Biol Inf* 1988;1:27–30.

Chapter 10

1. I Gerhard, F Postneek, "Auricular acupuncture in the treatment of female infertility," *Gynecol Endocrinol* 1992;6(3):171–181.

2. I Gerhard, F Postneek, "[Possibilities of therapy by ear acupuncture in female sterility]," *Geburtshilfe Frauenheilkd* 1988;48(3):165–171.

3. X Mo, D Li, Y Pu, et al., "Clinical studies on the mechanism for acupuncture stimulation of ovulation," *J Tradit Chin Med* 1993;13(2):115–119.

4. Paulus, et al., "Influence of acupuncture on the pregnancy rate in patients who undergo assisted reproduction therapy," *Fertility and Sterility* 2002;77(4).

5. R Riegler, F Fischl, et al., "[Correlation of psychological changes and spermiogram improvements following acupuncture]," *Urologe A* 1984;23(6):329–333.

6. S Siterman, F Eltes, et al., "Effect of acupuncture on sperm parameters of males suffering from subfertility related to low sperm quality," *Arch Androl* 1997;39(2):155–161.

7. Z Zheng, "Analysis on the therapeutic effect of combined use of acupuncture and medication in 297 cases of male sterility," *J Tradit Chin Med* 1997;17(3):190–193.

8. S Siterman, F Eltes, et al., "Does acupuncture treatment affect sperm density in males with very low sperm count? A pilot study," *Andrologia* 2000;32(1):31–39.

9. F Lian, "TCM treatment of luteal phase defect—an analysis of 60 cases," *J Tradit Chin Med* 1991;11(2):115–120.

10. HY Zhang, XZ Yu, GL Wang, "[Preliminary report of the treatment of luteal phase defect by replenishing kidney. An analysis of 53 cases]," *Zhongguo Zhong Xi Yi Jie He Za Zhi* 1992;12(8):473–474.

11. JX Liu, "[Clinical study of the treatment of endometriosis with traditional Chinese medicine]," *Zhongguo Zhong Xi Yi Jie He Za Zhi* 1994;14(6):337–339.

12. DZ Wang, ZQ Wang, ZF Zhang, "[Treatment of endometriosis with removing blood stasis and purgation method]," *Zhong Xi Yi Jie He Za Zhi* 1991;11(9):524–526.

13. D Tian, X Xie, B Wang, "[Study on relationship between ovulation inducing effect of drug-acupuncture and endometrial contents of estradiol receptor and progesterone receptor]," *Zhongguo Zhong Xi Yi Jie He Za Zhi* 1998;18(4):225–226.

14. DJ Li, CJ Li, Y Zhu, "[Treatment of immunological infertility with Chinese medicinal herbs of ziyin jianghuo]," *Zhongguo Zhong Zi Yi Jie He Za Zhi* 1995;15(1):3–5.

15. GP Yue, Q Chen, N Dai, "[Eighty-seven cases of male infertility treated by Bushen Shengjing Pill in clinical observation and evaluation on its curative effect]," *Zhongguo Zhong Zi Yi Jie He Za Zhi* 1996;16(8):463–466.

16. H Ishikawa, M Ohashi, et al., "Effects of guizhi-fuling-wan on male infertility with varicocele," *Am J Chin Med* 1996;24(3–4):327–331.

17. H Yoshida, T Tanifuji, et al., "[Clinical effects of Chinese herb medicine (Hochu-ekki-to) on infertile men]," *Hinyokika Kiyo* 1986;32(2):297–302.

18. S Usuki, "Hachimijiogan changes serum hormonal circumstance and improves spermatogenesis in oligozoospermic men," *Am J Chin Med* 1986;14(1–2):37–45.

19. A Okuyama, M Namiki, et al., "[Effects of Hachimijiogan and Ninjintoh on fertility in males with sterility]," *Hinyokika Kiyo* 1984;30(3):409–413.

20. H Takayama, T Konishi, et al., "[Clinical effects of Goshajinkigan for male infertility]," *Hinyokika Kiyo* 1984;30(11):1685–1689.

Chapter 11

1. L Long, E Ernst, "Homeopathic remedies for the treatment of osteoarthritis: A systematic review," *Br Homeopath J* 2001;90(1):37–43.

2. M Wiesenauer, "Comparison of solid and liquid forms of homeopathic remedies for tonsillitis," *Adv Ther* 1998;15(6):362–371.

3. I Gerhar, E Wallis, "Individualized homeopathic therapy for male infertility," *Homeopathy* 2002;91(3):133–144.

Index

About the Authors

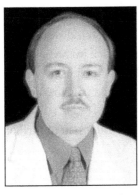

Chris D. Meletis, N.D., is a physician and educator whose life mission is to "change the world's health one person at a time." He has sought to fulfill his life's journey by becoming an educator of physicians, pharmacists, allied healthcare providers, and the general public, while at the same time seeing patients.

Dr. Meletis is an internationally published author, with ten books to his name and two pending publication. He has also contributed to another seven books and to dozens of national publications. As a regular columnist for professional journals, he routinely authors columns for the pharmacist and physician in such publications as *Natural Pharmacy* and the *Journal of Complementary and Alternative Medicine.* He has also had articles featured in such magazines as *Natural Health* and *Bottom Line Health.*

Over the years Dr. Meletis has sought to reach the public through regular radio programs such as *Scientific Nutrition, Back to the Beginning,* and *The Golden Radio Hour,* an Oregon Public Broadcasting series. He has been a guest on countless radio programs nationwide and throughout Canada, often reaching listening audiences of upwards of a million listeners at a time. Dr. Meletis has also been featured on several television programs focusing on natural medicine in the new millennium. As an educator Dr. Meletis lectures routinely to the medical community for continuing education on various natural medicine topics and safe use of natural products. He also enjoys giving talks to the public; one of his most recent presentations was as a panelist discussing the use of integrated medicine to an audience of over 1,200 women in conjunction with the local medical school in Portland, Oregon.

Dr. Meletis has also served as the Dean of Naturopathic Medicine and Chief Medical Officer at the National College of Naturopathic Medicine in Portland,

Oregon, for seven years. He now serves the NCNM as Senior Science Officer and Associate Professor of Natural Pharmacology. He has taught and continues to teach courses focusing on nutrition and nutraceutical and natural pharmacology, with an emphasis on using natural medicines as supported by the medical and scientific literature. In his academic and administrative role, Dr. Meletis helped create strategic alliances within the Portland metropolitan area, including setting up twelve community clinics for NCNM physicians, students, and residents to provide patient care annually to some 12,000 patients who are low income and homeless and who otherwise would go without healthcare. Dr. Meletis also was named the 2003 Naturopathic Physician of the Year by the American Association of Naturopathic Physicians (AANP), the profession's national organization.

As a consultant to the healthcare industry, Dr. Meletis has served in numerous capacities, including product formulator, technical advisor, research director, and vice president of medical affairs. He believes that natural medicine in the new millennium must "blend the best of nature and science" and that individuals need to seek the best attributes of all forms of healthcare to achieve and maintain optimal health.

Dr. Meletis has a website available to the public for those interested in further health information: www.divinemedicine.com.

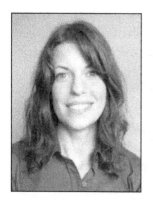 **Liz Brown** is a health and nutrition writer based in Portland, Oregon. She earned a bachelor's of science degree in nutrition from the University of Minnesota, Twin Cities, and contributes regularly to consumer magazines, newspapers, and books on topics of health, with a special interest in natural and preventive medicine and nutritional anthropology. Her articles have appeared in such magazines as *Better Nutrition, Great-Life, Natural Pharmacy, Physical,* and *Spa,* among others. Brown is also coauthor, with Jack Challem, of *Basic Health Publications User's Guide to Vitamins and Minerals,* published in 2002.

www.ingramcontent.com/pod-product-compliance
Lightning Source LLC
Jackson TN
JSHW011400130125
77033JS00023B/775